Alzheimer's disease: Beyond the medical model

edited by
Matthew V Morrissey and Ann-Louise Coakley

Quay
Books

Mark Allen
Publishing Ltd

Quay Books Division, Mark Allen Publishing Ltd, Jesses Farm,
Snow Hill, Dinton, Salisbury, Wiltshire SP3 5HN

British Library Cataloguing-in-Publication Data
A catalogue record for this book is available from the British Library

ISBN 1 85642 095 7
© Mark Allen Publishing 1999

Printed in the United Kingdom by The Cromwell Press, Trowbridge,
Wiltshire

Contents

Acknowledgements

Many people have assisted in the preparation of this text. We cannot name everyone but would like to extend our warmest thanks to:

- The Alzheimer's Disease Society
- Nursing students at Canterbury Christ Church University College, Canterbury, Kent
- Clarecastle Women's Fund Raising Care Group, County Clare, Ireland
- Carers' Group, Darland House, Gillingham, Kent
- All the staff at Frank Lloyd Home, Sittingbourne, Paul Guppy, Syd Peerbux, Patricia Potter
- Peter Marsh and staff at Southlands Ward, Keycol Hospital
- Sittingbourne, All Saints CPN Service, Chatham, Kent
- Staff at the Day Hospital Memorial Hospital, Sittingbourne, Kent
- James, Elizabeth and Claire Robinson, Matthew and Mary, Kenneth and Valerie, Jennifer and Nicole Chantelle, Sonya, Kevin, Fiona and Paudy, Darragh and Cian
- Special thanks to Valerie Marston and Tamzin, Binkie and Caroline.

Special thanks to families and friends for their patience and support in this creative project. Any errors or omissions are those of the respective authors and the views expressed by authors are not necessarily those of their employing organisations.

Matthew V Morrissey and Ann-Louise Coakley
Faculty of Nursing, Midwifery and Social Work
Canterbury Christ Church University College
January, 1999

List of Contributors

Ann-Louise Coakley is a senior lecturer and research coordinator in the Faculty of Nursing, Midwifery and Social Work at Canterbury Christ Church University College and an experienced researcher in the field of healthcare.

David T Evans is a senior lecturer in sociology at the University of Glasgow. He has published a number of articles on sociology. His writings about sexuality include *Sexual Citizenship: The Material Construction of Sexualities* (Routledge, 1993).

Robert-Gareth Hill previously a research associate with the Sainsbury Centre for Mental Health. Presently undertaking a doctorate in clinical psychology. Research interests include philosophy, manic depression, existential psychology and mental health.

Mary Morrissey is chair and driving force behind a fund raising project that has provided one of the largest day care centres in County Clare, Ireland. The centre provides day care and respite care for people with dementia. Her main interests relate to the improvement of care for older people, their relatives and carers.

Matthew V Morrissey is a senior lecturer (in mental health) at Canterbury Christ Church University College. His research interests include mental health, human rights, Alzheimer's disease and elderly care, and sexuality and healthcare.

Elizabeth Robinson is a senior lecturer (nursing and midwifery) at Canterbury Christ Church University College.

James Robinson is a solicitor working in child protection and mental health legal services with Kent County Council.

Jane Webborn is a senior nurse at Ty Hafan Children's Hospital in Wales and has particular interest in grief and loss in relation to the family unit.

Preface

Caring for a person with Alzheimer's disease and dementia is the most challenging aspect of elderly care. There is no definitive text on how to care but the focus of care needs to move beyond the medical model and into the arena of care in its broadest sense. For carers and nurses the work is exhausting on many levels. Frequently there is a lack of resources, education and support and the ever-changing pattern of work often means leadership is weak. Some elderly care homes fail to recognise psychological and social aspects of care due to the enormous demands of physical care. Cases of dementia and Alzheimer's disease are happening to younger and younger people.

Alzheimer's disease makes incredible demands on relatives and care staff and the effects of such care can have negative consequences. The greatest injustice is that little recognition or support is given to carers, nursing and other support staff. Like Tom Kitwood who has pioneered work in dementia, this book continues to affirm the person and personal aspects of a person with Alzheimer's disease rather than simply viewing the person as someone to be handed over and treated by a medical model. The text combines a critical approach to theory and practice. It is compiled as a textbook for healthcare professionals, for carers, nurses and those studying courses in healthcare and related subjects.

There has been a substantial development in degree and post-graduate courses in nursing and healthcare. Intrinsic to many of these is the need to study elderly care, and more specifically care related to dementia and Alzheimer's disease. Not only do healthcare workers need to understand issues relating to this area, but increasingly they need to have knowledge and skills in practice. Furthermore, there is a need to develop policy in many areas where the person with Alzheimer's disease is affected, both directly and indirectly, by healthcare practices.

The text offers a collection of perspectives which promote the understanding of those issues surrounding the care of a person with Alzheimer's disease. Healthcare workers are frequently involved in decisions about care and need to feel comfortable and be conversant with issues surrounding Alzheimer's disease.

Matthew V Morrissey

Overview

Dementing disorders are unfortunately the most common disorders of later life and are linked to medical, social and economic problems to name but a few. This book aims to expose the reader to the various aspects of Alzheimer's disease that have impact not only on sufferers themselves but on those who care for them. The book is divided into two parts; *Part One* deals with the real meaning of care and in *PartTwo* the psychological and practical aspects of care are explored.

In *Chapter One*, Matthew Morrissey examines current issues in care including diagnosis, drug therapy, support for caregivers and professional attitudes to elderly care. He emphasises the growing dissatisfaction with the so-called 'medical model' of care and the need for a wider, more 'loving' perspective to be provided. In *Chapter Two*, Robert Hill discusses the way to a greater understanding of what Alzheimer's disease means to carers. He also underlines the potential influence of the way in which we talk about the disease and how this affects the process of care and the disease trajectory. The first part of the book is concluded with a chapter by David Evans who examines the sociological background to Alzheimer's disease and the way in which cultural communication, social interaction, media interpretation and the narratives of all the key players shape our understanding of the disease.

Part Two begins with a chapter by Matthew Morrissey, describing the loss and bereavement experienced by carers and their families. He suggests ways in which management of the disease and support for carers could be improved and includes the way in which Alzheimer's disease in a relative or friend affects children. In *Chapter Five*, James Robinson and Matthew Morrissey examine the legal and financial issues that Alzheimer's disease raises and offer advice on the best ways of dealing with any problems that arise, including power of attorney and the role of 'the nearest relative'. The book concludes with a chapter detailing experiences of care by carers themselves. There is a moving account by Mary Morrissey of the way in which her own initial lack of knowledge about Alzheimer's disease frustrated her ability to care for her mother. Jane Webborn plots the path of Alzheimer's in a relative and shows graphically how Alzheimer's has drained relatives and friends. The third narrative comes from Elizabeth Robinson who describes 'Linda's story', including the experience of assessment and, eventually, compulsory admission to hospital. The final narrative is anonymous, but highlights again the impact of the disease on relatives and, in particular, the difficulties of balancing other family needs and a reasonable life for carers.

The last section of the book, the *Appendix*, provides some useful contact addresses for carers of people with Alzheimer's, including those of the Alzheimer's Disease Society and its branches.

The editors hope this book, will open the door to new ways of thinking about Alzheimer's disease and, at the very least, stimulate debate between all those involved in care.

Ann-Louise Coakley

Part 1:
The meaning of care

1
Current issues in care

Matthew V Morrissey

There are millions of people world wide with Alzheimer's disease and a growing elderly population. Close to the heart of many carers and nurses is the desire to provide care which is humane and protects the dignity of the person.

(Matthew V Morrissey, 1999)

Issues in care

At present there is no cure, successful treatment or prevention method for Alzheimer's disease. There is also the growing problem of trying to provide care for younger and younger people with dementia (Morgan and Stewart, 1999; Keady and Matthew, 1997). There are millions of people world wide with Alzheimer's disease and a growing elderly population. Close to the heart of many carers and nurses is the desire to provide care which is humane and protects the dignity of the person. Clearly medical care is essential, but it is time that the voices of carers and nurses and other health professionals is expressed so that they can be involved in present and future initiatives in care.

There is a growing dissatisfaction with the traditional medical model. Such an approach tends to dominate practice and excludes other approaches in caring for the person with dementia. We need to understand that a medical model alone fails to define and understand nursing, psychology, emotional and spiritual care. It is vital that we become conscious of the intense human suffering around Alzheimer's disease beyond the physical realm, and also vital we are alert to abuse (Ogg and Bennett, 1992). In its past history and in the present too, the medical model and the practice of medicine have rarely grappled with the emotional and psychological aspects of care. Such aspects were often seen as peripheral and patients as a series of procedures. It is time to shift the focus of dementia care so that results can be measured in improved quality of care, respect, comfort and team work.

When evaluating current approaches to medical research, can we be sure that medicine is asking the right questions for the person dependent on its care? Recent approaches have helped to educate relatives and carers and have explored Alzheimer's disease from the client's perspective (Greenway and Walker, 1998).

The medical model is frequently more concerned in the outcome than the process. For the most part, doctors tend to focus on the clinical and the physical domains and, in the later stages of dementia, the person may be viewed simply as a body. It seems there is a reluctance to engage in research which can empower people in care. Tom Kitwood, a pioneer in this area, stressed the importance of 'person-hood', and in his book, *Dementia Reconsidered,* he too questions the medical model and also recognises the barrier that the power and prestige of the medical profession poses (Kitwood, 1997).

Dementia has traditionally been presented as the proper territory for psychiatry, with the implication that all other disciplines should defer to its 'higher' knowledge. Indeed, there is a view that people with dementia owe to society the offering of themselves for research as a form of payment for their care (Berghmans and ter Meulen, 1995; Kitwood, 1997).

Alzheimer's disease: the facts

Alzheimer's disease is an incurable neurological disease in which changes in the nerve cells of the brain result in brain degeneration and eventually brain death. The destruction of brain cells eventually gives rise to serious mental deterioration, mental health problems, dementia and death.

Presently the majority of carers in the UK are women (Parker *et al*, 1996; Nankervis *et al*, 1997). However, this pattern is changing as more and more women go out to work and extended family support becomes a rarity (Pickles, 1998). To date the focus of much of the research is in the neuroscience field (Jones and Mimieson, 1993) and little research exists in the area of dementia care. It has been clear for many years that there is a genetic connection in some cases of Alzheimer's disease, namely an abnormality on chromosome 21 which results in Downs syndrome. More recently, in 1995, the discovery of chromosome 14 showed the specific gene responsible for the familial early onset of Alzheimer's disease.

With such discoveries, many families are asking whether or not they can be tested for their risk of developing Alzheimer's disease. At present the APOE4 gene is a risk factor, but it is not possible even to state the exact degree of risk it confers (Gunnarsson and Lundberg, 1995). Clearly, even if there were a full proof test, a minefield of legal, social, personal, and ethical issues would still arise.

More importantly, the link between genetics and treatment may be poles apart. What do we do until they find the miracle cure? How will we provide care for the increasing elderly population and, specifically, the millions with Alzheimer's disease?

The Government's social trends survey in the UK predicts that the number of people over 65 will rise from 9 million to 12 million over the next 30 years (Pickles, 1998). Figures for dementia will also increase and at least half of these could have Alzheimer's disease. In America between about 4 million to 6.8 million people have dementia (Office of Technology Assessment, 1990). However, a more recent study in the UK indicates that the incidence of dementia and Alzheimer's disease rises exponentially up to the age of 90 years, with no sign of levelling off. Women were also found to have a higher incidence of Alzheimer's disease in very old age, and men tended to have a higher incidence of vascular dementia at younger ages (Jorm and Jolley, 1998).

In a Dutch study it was concluded that the application of an individualised cut-off for the screening instrument resulted in the detection of a substantial number of cases with very mild dementia, which subsequently resulted in higher incidence rates than those reported in most other studies (Anderson *et al*, 1999). By the middle of the twenty-first century, the number diagnosed with Alzheimer's in America may reach 14 million. Alzheimer's is the fourth leading cause of death in adults, preceded only by heart disease, cancer and stroke. It is estimated that one in ten families has a member who has Alzheimer's disease (Dittbrenner, 1994; Nadler-Moodie and Foltz-Wilson, 1998).

Alzheimer's disease most commonly affects individuals who are over 65, however, it can also affect people much younger. About 11 per cent of all Americans over 65, and 25 to 50 per cent of those over 85, are believed to have the disease.

Statistically, Alzheimer's disease represents almost half of the total population described as having senile dementia. People with Alzheimer's disease occupy more than half the beds in skilled nursing facilities (Morgan and Stewart, 1998).

Diagnosis

Diagnosis of Alzheimer's disease is achieved by ruling out other diseases with similar symptoms such as brain tumours, strokes and infections. The clinician must also discount the occasional forgetfulness that occurs during normal ageing and other factors such as malnutrition or depression, as these conditions can mimic Alzheimer's-like memory loss. To be effective with a diagnosis, clinicians must be expert in this area and use sound clinical evaluation, for there continues to be no accurate diagnostic laboratory test for Alzheimer's disease.

Ideally a diagnosis is established after thorough medical evaluation followed by both extensive neurological and neuropsychological assessments, but a definitive diagnosis can be made only by an autopsy. During the first couple of years, individuals with Alzheimer's disease usually have problems with short-term memory; that is, they experience memory loss for recent events. Disorientation is not uncommon and very often the individual will have some problems with progressive memory loss, judgement, basic maths, perception, speech and language comprehension, and also physical co-ordination.

Basic housework and other routines such as bathing and toileting often present the individual and family with problems. As time goes on and Alzheimer's disease takes a firm hold, the individual's family or carer will probably have to provide full-time supervision because the person will have a tendency to wander off and sometimes to engage in antisocial behaviour. Indeed, many more behaviours may cause problems for others as the person become less aware of self and others, and conflict is sometimes the result. Other behaviours include 'fiddling', and collecting and misplacing objects. Sadly, self-care becomes impossible and the person eventually becomes almost totally dependent on carers.

Other common problems include sleeplessness marked by anxious agitation in the evening and perseveration which means the sometimes continuous repetition of the same ideas, words, movements or thoughts. The most severe and final stage as the disease progresses includes significant problems with eating, communication and control of body functions. However, there are also difficult behaviour problems to contend with. Emotions such as irritability and anger, as well as stubbornness and obnoxiousness are not uncommon. Unfortunately behavioural problems are part of the disease; they are not malicious but may be perceived as such unless there is awareness of the condition.

The so-called group of 'six Rs' put forward by Nancy Mace and Peter Rabins, is one way of dealing with difficult behaviour. In simplicity, this involves managing the behaviour of a person by Restricting, Reassessing, Reconsidering, Re-channelling, Reassurance and Reviewing each behaviour (Mace and Rabins, 1991).

Treatment

Drug therapy

The drugs used for dementia, and more particularly for Alzheimer's disease, include Donepezil, Tacrine and ENA-713 which are all acetylcholinesterase inhibitors. These drugs increase the availability of acetylcholine, a neurotransmitter needed for memory and learning.

It has been suggested that in the early stages these drugs may lessen the cognitive signs and symptoms and slow the progression of the disease (Nadler-Moodie and Foltz-Wilson, 1998). However, other reports challenge such benefits (Feely, 1997). At the present time there is no way to prevent or cure Alzheimer's disease. In 1993, Tacrine (Cognex) was approved in the US and is now widely available by prescription from general practitioners. The medication requires blood tests every two weeks for the first 18 weeks of administration to check for liver inflammation, a common side effect.

Results of studies on Tacrine have shown it to be of modest benefit in a minority of patients. It does not stop the progression of the illness but may provide symptomatic improvement in a small number of patients. Patients and family members are encouraged to discuss such treatments with their physician or general practitioner. Other drugs are also under study to examine their efficacy and safety in treating Alzheimer's disease.

These 'other drugs' include DHEA and oestrogen which are hormones, and anti-inflammatory medications such as Prednisolone, all of which are aimed at treating entirely different causes of the disease. In addition, there are current experimental drug trials looking at the treatment of agitated behaviours using both pharmacological and behavioural approaches.

Comprehensive treatment, if available, must address the needs of the entire family. This should include emotional support, counselling and educational courses about Alzheimer's disease for patients and family members. Respite care is essential and home help is often required. Day care is frequently an essential ingredient in support, as is legal and financial advice.

Managing the agitation and distress of individuals with Alzheimer's disease can be very difficult. Recently, multi-sensory environments have been employed to help with such behaviours, with some positive consequences (Baker *et al*,1997; Morrissey and Biela, 1997). A randomised controlled trial was employed in the study by Baker and colleagues (Baker *et al*, 1997). The long-term benefits of Snoezelen were in the domain of socially disturbed behaviour. Short-term improvements in behaviour and mood were evident for both groups after sessions, and communication was significantly better during Snoezelen sessions in comparison with activity sessions.

Support for caregivers

There is now much research to show that when spouses join support groups and receive counselling to help them to cope with the effect of their partners' symptoms, their partners fare better and remain at home longer (Collins *et al*, 1994). Caregivers who participate in awareness training and problem-solving programmes are better able to manage difficult behaviours such as wandering, hoarding and inappropriate sexual behaviour (Ghatak, 1994).

However, counselling and support are not available for many due to lack of resources (Kitwood, 1997). It is important both to explain to and inform relatives and family about the nature and progression of Alzheimer's disease. It is also important to explore individuals' emotional and psychological reactions to the deterioration of their relative.

Education is crucial and it is often helpful to suggest certain texts or to provide handouts. Some care homes have their own courses which may include education for children and adolescents. Families may need help in finding support and new coping strategies; such aid is sometimes part of a service run by voluntary groups.

Attitudes of professionals to elderly care

> *Suffer us not to mock ourselves with falsehood*
> *Teach us to care and not to care*
> *Teach us to sit still*

(Ash Wednesday, TS Eliot)

Elderly care has never been truly valued by medicine, as is reflected in attitudes towards geriatric medicine which consider it to be 'a second rate speciality, looking after third rate patients, in fourth rate facilities' (BMA, 1986).

There lies a vulnerability between service and personal advantage, a wrenching vulnerability felt when one partner goes into full-time care sometimes leaving the partner, who is often the carer, alone. Certain occupations profess to love, claiming both the title 'profession' and a commitment to service of mankind. These groups are both professors and lovers it seems. Indeed, what they profess in addition to knowledge and skill, is disinterested love (Campbell, 1984). They are set apart from other occupational groups, including other professions, by being described as 'welfare professions', 'caring professions'. 'They promise to deliver not just physical treatment or material aid but a tenderness (which) absorbs manipulation' (Halmos, 1965). They also profess to deal with people in a way not simply based on the rules of fair trading but also on an ethic of 'respect for persons'.

The word 'love' is rarely, if ever, used by doctors, nurses, or social workers themselves to describe their professional relationships with clients or patients. In fact, in psychotherapy and counselling psychology there seems some great virtue in remaining detached from the client. Such an approach to care is clearly not appropriate or sufficient for the nursing care of people with Alzheimer's disease.

A cure for Alzheimer's is still a distant dream in spite of various recent claims in the media (Zinser, 1998). Recognising this, the real focus must move towards care beyond a medical model whose main obsession is finding cures. Neuroscientific research dominates the headlines, overshadowing the advances made in care-giving (Jones and Mimieson, 1993). We must also realise how important hope is to all involved in care, a view also expressed by Kitwood (1997). Care continues to be dominated by medical interventions and drugs whose efficacy could easily be contested given recent reports by doctors (Feely, 1997).

Information about Alzheimer's disease is often accessed at a late stage in the provision of care, resulting in many carers being deprived of much-needed understanding and support earlier on. In the next chapters, issues related to care will be explored which will help to show how we need to care beyond the medical model if we are to deliver care to a person, not a disease.

References

Andersen K, Nielsen H, Lolk A *et al* (1999) Incidence of very mild dementia and Alzheimer's disease in Denmark: The Odense Study. *Neurology* **52**(1): 85–90

Baker R, Dowling Z, Wareing LA *et al* (1997) Snoezelen: Its long-term and short-term effects on older people with dementia. *Br J Occ Ther* **60**(5): 213–7

Berghmans RLP, ter Meulen RHJ (1995) Ethical issues in research with dementia patients. *Int J Ger Psychiatry* **10**: 647–51

British Medical Association (1986) *All our tomorrows: growing old in Britain.* BMA, London

Campbell AV (1984) *Moderated Love: A Theology of Professional Care.* Holy Trinity Church, Marylebone Road, London

Collins C, Stommel M, Wang S *et al* (1994) Caregiving transitions: changes in depression among family caregivers of relatives with dementia. *Nurs Res* **43**(4): 220–5

Dittbrenner H (1994) Alzheimer's disease: the long goodbye. *Caring Mag* Aug: 14–23

Eliot TS (1969) *Complete Poems and Plays.* Faber & Faber, London

Feely J (1997) Alzheimer's Disease. *Health Which?*: 172–3

Ghatak R (1994) Effects of an intervention programme on dementia patients and the caregivers. *Caring Magazine* Aug: 34–9

Greenway M, Walker A (1998) Home health. Helping caregivers cope with Alzheimer's disease. *Nursing* **28**(2):1–2, 4–6

Gunnarson LG, Lundberg C (1995) Cautiousness in testing for Alzheimer's disease. *Am J Alzheimer Dis* Jul/Aug: 37–8

Halmos P (1965) *The Faith of the Counsellors.* Constable, London

Jones G, Mimieson B (1993) *Care-giving in Dementia.* Routledge, London

Jorm A, Jolly D (1998) The incidence of dementia: a meta-analysis. *Neurology* **51**(3): 728–33

Keady J, Matthew L (1997) Younger people with dementia. *Elderly Care* **9**(4):19–23

Kitwood T (1997) *Dementia Reconsidered.* Open University Press

Mace N, Rabins P (1991) *The 36 Hour Day.* The John Hopkins University Press, Baltimore, Maryland, USA

Morgan DG, Stewart NJ (1998) Multiple occupancy versus private rooms on dementia care units. *Environ Behav* **30**(4): 487–503

Morgan DG, Stewart NJ (1999) The physical environment of special care units: Needs of residents with dementia from the perspective of staff and family caregivers. *Qualitative Health Res* **9**(1): 105–18

Morrissey M, Biela C (1997) Care of older people. Sneozelen: benefits for nursing older clients *Nurs Stand* **12**(3):38–40

Nadler-Moodie M, Foltz-Wilson (1998) Latest approaches in Alzheimer's care. *Registered Nurse* **61**(7): 42–6

Office of Technology Assessment, US Congress (1990) *Confused Minds, Burdened Families.* US Government Printing Office, Washington DC

Ogg J, Bennett G (1992) Elder Abuse in Britain. *Br Med J* **305**(24): 998–9

Parker G, Scazufca M, Kuipers E (1996) Women as carers of the severely mentally ill. In: Abel K, Buszewicz M, eds. *et al* (1996) *Planning community mental health services for women. A multiprofessional handbook.* Routledge, London

Pickles H (1998) Caring for the elderly: part two. You're not born to sacrifice your life to look after your parents. *You Magazine, Mail on Sunday*, Associated Newspapers Ltd, London, June: 42–7

Zinser S (1998) 'A drug that can give Alzheimer's sufferers a brainpower boost'. Daily Mail, July: 28, 45

2

Where is the life we have lost in living? The search for personal meaning in Alzheimer's disease

Robert Gareth Hill

The meaning of life is from within us, it is not bestowed from without, and it far exceeds in both its beauty and permanence any heaven of which men have ever dreamed or yearned for.

(Taylor, 1987)

O wondrous change! Those hands, once so strong and active, have now been bound. Helpless and forlorn, you see the end of your deed. Yet with a sigh of relief you resign your cause to a stronger hand, and are content to do so. For one brief moment you enjoyed the bliss of freedom, only to give it back to God, that he might perfect it in glory.

(Bonhoeffer, 1959)

Introduction

It is one of the cruel facts of Alzheimer's disease that one knows what awaits the individual at the end of a long and painful process. This is probably true at some point for both the person with the condition and their carers and loved ones. Unlike many diseases, although similar to some, there is no choice of destination and, at most, a limited choice about how one arrives. Research into the disease has even managed to provide a timetable of quite devastating accuracy, with death usually occurring within five to eight years (Gelder *et al*, 1996). Such pronouncements take on an almost cryptic quality as if they were 'magic' numbers, but we know they aren't really 'magic' because, unlike 'magic', they take everything away without ever giving anything back. Why, it is legitimate to ask, after all the suffering is there such a predictable and final outcome? As Viktor Frankl (1959) states, 'to those things that seem to take meaning away from human life belong not only suffering but dying as well, not only distress but also death.' Given such an undeniable outcome, where is meaning itself to be located? For some people the end point will undoubtedly supply the meaning, whether this is seen as liberation from affliction, 'peace at last' or a higher movement into another less tangible but more important form of reality. For others the end is paradoxically the beginning of the search for meaning, a way of understanding how a valuable life could be 'spoilt' by not achieving all that lay before it. Others still will have found answers during the process of care; death being the natural outcome of a process with which they came to terms, often on a daily basis.

The 'burden' of caring

Of the many books written for those who care for someone with Alzheimer's disease, questions of carer 'burden' and coping loom understandably large. 'Burden' has been described as the presence of problems, difficulties or adverse events which affect the life (lives)' of a person's significant others (Platt, 1985). It is now commonplace to distinguish between 'objective' burdens and 'subjective' burdens. 'Objective burden' is used to identify 'anything that occurs as a disrupting factor in family life owing to the patient's illness' (Hoening, 1968), while 'subjective burden' refers to the feeling that a burden is being carried by an individual in a very personal and private way (Hoening and Hamilton, 1967). Those areas of difficulty commonly associated with caring for someone with Alzheimer's disease have been categorised into four main areas: practical problems; behavioural problems; interpersonal problems; and social problems (Levin *et al*, 1989).

Mace *et al* (1988), in their book *The 36-Hour Day*, examine these areas from a practical standpoint, and it is easy to understand how such difficulties may contribute to the 15 per cent or so of carers who themselves become clinically depressed. Thus, it is important to consider practical ways of helping those who care for someone with Alzheimer's disease. Levin (1991), cited in Gelder *et al*, (1996), for instance, recommends the following key requirements when thinking about providing comprehensive support for carers.

1   Early identification of dementia (the role of general practitioners is vital).

2   Comprehensive medical and social assessment of identified cases.

3   Timely referrals between agencies, for example from GP to old-age psychiatrist.
4   Continuing reviews of each patient's needs and backup for carers.
5   Active medical treatment for any other illnesses present;
6   the provision of information, advice and counselling for carers.
7   Regular help with household and personal tasks.
8   Regular breaks for carers, for example by providing day care and respite care for patients.
9   Appropriate financial support.
10   Permanent residential care when this becomes necessary.

Understandably, the level of strain and burden experienced by carers relates to the mechanisms they develop in order to cope. As Burns *et al* (1995) note:

> *Several types of coping have been described. One distinction which has been made is that between behavioural (active commissioning of help) and psychological (internal readjustment) coping. Responses to the stress of coping consist of those attempting to change the situation, those controlling the meaning of the stressful event and those which control stress by changing the interpretation of stress into a moral virtue (e.g. individuals saying they have a duty to look after their relatives).*

(Burns *et al*, 1995)

This distinction between changing the situation and changing the interpretation is an important one, and one that is increasingly being used in psychological therapies such as cognitive-behaviour therapy. Such therapies usefully remind us that we don't simply react to events in the world but that it is the interpretations we make of the events that are often more significant. Such interpretations inevitably tend to occur within the context of how we already see the world and how we understand our place within it.

This chapter is about how we may come to understand Alzheimer's disease and the meaning we may give to something that on the surface seems so cruel and purposeless. Kushner (1981), writing about the experience of Alzheimer's disease, uses the memorable phrase 'bad things happen to good people' as the title for the book. Unlike other chapters in this book, this one may seem to be less practically focused.

In one sense this is true, indeed it is the central proposition of this chapter that questions of meaning have been excluded from a great deal of the literature on Alzheimer's disease. Moreover, the ways in which Alzheimer's disease is discussed by clinicians, the ways in which the media represent the disease and the ways in which we talk about it, do not necessarily fulfil all of the needs of those who care or have a personal relationship with someone with Alzheimer's disease.

In intent, this chapter is concerned with carers and professionals communicating with each other about what it truly means to have Alzheimer's disease. It is not practical in the sense that it is not about saying what things *should* mean, for meaning is something that is derived out of relationships and personal beliefs. At another level, though, the search for meaning provides the basis for action and if there is any doubt as to the importance of meaning in our lives, I would simply quote Schrum (1989):

> *Life is lived according to meaning. How we respond to a situation, relationship, or idea will depend on what it means to us. Numberless meanings fill both the culture of society and the life of each one of us, shaping intentions, guiding actions, and evaluating results, but behind this unending array there lies one particular which is central and which everywhere reaches out to penetrate the rest — it is the sense of meaning to our life as a whole. Within it we find the essential challenge in the field of meaning: to discover in the entirety of our living, meaning that is deep and true.*

(Schrum, 1989)

This chapter is also about society's representation of Alzheimer's disease; a representation that is intimately tied to perceptions of the elderly generally. Whether people have a specified illness or are 'just being' looked after, what tends to be neglected is the wider question of personal meaning; a question that is fundamental to our lives as human beings. Carers are more than the politicians' 'surrogate professionals' or the media's 'saints' and 'sinners' and where such language is used, the importance of the personal relationship is undeniably overlooked. One person responding to another with a disease is not the same as one person responding to another person. John Bayley's (1998) moving account of his relationship with his wife, Iris Murdoch, is a good example of this.

The burden of meaning

Even though meaning is central to our lives it is an area about which we remain curiously silent. Gerontologists and others who study old age can explain all about the organic pathology of the damaged brain in as simple or complex terms as the hearer requires, and other health professionals will talk about the course of the illness and offer practical suggestions about care and advice on personal coping strategies. The media, when focusing on Alzheimer's disease generally, focus on scientific and medical breakthroughs interspersed with individual case studies. What they tend not to focus on is the question of what it means either to have Alzheimer's disease or to look after someone with the disease. In other words, there is generally no attempt to focus on questions of understanding, purpose and intent. It is as if this is the one subject that would be too painful to bear; almost as if the physical and mental deterioration of a loved one or other important person is bearable just so long as we don't ask why. Why her? Why him? Why now? Why at all? Moreover, this silence as to meaning is not the comfortable silence of acceptance but a deafening silence; a silence of discomfort, a silence which, undoubtedly with good intentions, we all share. Yet it is these questions about meaning that are at the centre of our being. It is these questions that keep us awake, even if it is more practical concerns that keep us from sleep.

We set professionals up to fail; we want them to have all the answers, even though we know that they don't. Professionals tend, and need, to think in practical terms, and engagement in questions of meaning may seem too abstruse and too far beyond their professional expertise to be important. Yet we also want professionals to talk to us at the level we all share: the shared level of being a distressed human being. One explanation for this silence has been suggested by Kitwood and Bredin (1992):

> *Professionals and informal carers are vulnerable people too, bearing their own anxiety and dread concerning frailty, dependency, madness, ageing, dying and death. A supposed objectivity in a context that is, in fact, interpersonal, is one way of maintaining psychological defences, and so making involvement with conditions such as dementia bearable.*

(Kitwood and Bredin, 1992)

What causes such basic difficulties? Is it because meaning is so very personal that we all implicitly agree not to talk about it or explore it? Is it because for all of us reading this now, Alzheimer's disease is a potentially yet-to-come experience? Or is it because, inevitably, the question of meaning leads on to the purpose of life and thence to death? Zygmunt Bauman (1992) notes that 'death (more exactly, awareness of mortality) is the ultimate condition of cultural creativity. It makes permanence into a task, into an urgent task, into a paramount task.' In other words, when such tasks cease or can no longer be fulfilled, we are left face to face with a destiny we had hoped to overcome. For the spectator in another's life, such an obvious confrontation with reality results in an inevitable raising of questions concerning the purpose of one's own life task, one's responsibilities towards others and one's own destiny. Moreover, this search for meaning is generally not fixed once and for all, but is always changing: as Schrum (1989) notes, 'to reconsider one's life is, at heart, clearly a daily concern, not something to have done and be done with doing.'

The tasks of life

One of the reasons for the devastating impact of Alzheimer's disease on carers is the recognition that what went before is not the same as what exists here and now. This is true of other illnesses and accidents, particularly individuals who sustain some form of brain injury as a result of traumatic head injury. But even this is too simple, for often the person we see before us and interact with, is both the same and different. On one level nothing has changed, at another everything. It is a confrontation with both repetition and difference. Thus, even where we feel a closeness to the person (wherein lie our feelings of moral responsibility) and we are less concerned with their identity, it is clear that their tasks of life have changed. Alzheimer's disease results in a different form of encounter with the world and with others, and probably with the self. It is, to use a crude simile, as if two actors become transformed into one actor and one director. Why, though, does this changed relationship to the world, self, and others matter? Richard Taylor (1987), in a paper entitled 'The Meaning of Life', puts it as follows:

> *A human being no sooner draws his first breath than he responds to the will that is in him to live. He no more asks whether it will be worthwhile, or whether anything of*

significance will come of it, than the worms and the birds. The point of his living is simply to be living, in the manner that it is his nature to be living. He goes through his life building his castles, each of these beginning to fade into time as the next is begun; yet, it would be no salvation to rest from all this. It would be a condemnation, and one that would in no way be redeemed were he able to gaze upon the things he has done, even if these were beautiful and absolutely permanent, as they never are. What counts is that one should be able to begin a new task, a new castle, a new bubble. It counts only because it is there to be done and he has the will to do it.

(Taylor, 1987)

What is so difficult about Alzheimer's disease is that the new castles and bubbles are not new at all, but merely old ones; everyday, taken-for-granted actions that previously were undertaken naturally. What was once a simple matter becomes an insoluble cryptic puzzle. With the progression of the illness, thought has to be directed consciously and behaviours that we felt had been learnt once and for all, become forever new. Falling off one's bike becomes an everyday reality to those with Alzheimer's disease. It is not the purpose of this chapter to examine such difficulties from the view of those with Alzheimer's disease. Many good accounts now exist — autobiographical (Davis, 1989; McGowin, 1993), relational (Bayley, 1998; Doerberg, 1989; Kushner, 1981) and academic (Goldsmith, 1996) — although it is fair to say that the internal perspective of the individual with Alzheimer's disease is a neglected area of research (Cotrell and Schulz, 1993). Moreover, while the search for meaning is crucial for carers, it is no less important that the individuals experiencing the symptoms of Alzheimer's should also be given the opportunity to understand the meaning of what is happening to them. An excellent and very moving account of just such an exploration through psychotherapy is to be found in Valerie Sinason's (1992) book.

Life itself can also be seen as a task following certain predictable stages, with illness as an unwanted disruption. Erikson's (1968) eight-stage developmental psycho-social theory views old age as a time of wisdom forged out of the search for meaning in the face of death. Whether such a view of a unified life course is correct, it is one that is embedded in the popular consciousness, and anything that stands in the way of such progress is seen as problematic. However, such development, while not exactly reversed, is viewed as irrelevant once someone reaches the designated and arbitrary time of old age. As Simone de Beauvoir (1972) states:

> *People have said to me, 'So long as you feel young, you are young.' This shows a complete misunderstanding of the complex truth of old age; for the outsider it is a dialectic relationship between my being as he defines it objectively and the awareness of myself that I acquire by means of him. Within me it is the Other — that is to say the person I am for the outsider — who is old, and the Other is myself.*

(de Beauvoir, 1972)

This is an important point and, before moving on, it is necessary to say something about how the old are perceived in society generally, for it is not easy to separate out negative views of the elderly generally from the negative stereotyping of Alzheimer's disease.

Representations of the old

> *I'm sorry about your mother's death. There was nothing that actually killed her except old age, but I'm not allowed to put that down as a cause of death on the death certificate, so I've put Alzheimer's disease down instead.*

(General practitioner)

My own grandmother was 103 years old when she died; a retired schoolteacher who had lived in her own house in the Welsh valleys until the age of 97. She was in charge of all her faculties when she died and there had never been any indication that she had any of the 'five As' associated with Alzheimer's disease: Amnesia (memory disturbance); Aphasia (word blindness); Apraxia (difficulty in undertaking a volitional act); Agnosia (inability to understand the significance of sensory stimuli) and Associated features such as psychiatric and behavioural disturbances (Burns *et al*, 1995). Indeed, up until her death she was reading a daily paper along with the *Reader's Digest*. Why, then, would the doctor who wrote the death certificate put Alzheimer's disease down as the cause of death? We do not know and, while it is important personally to find an answer to this question, the fact that a general practitioner can cite Alzheimer's disease as a cause of death, says a lot about how old people are perceived even by the well informed. Indeed, the doctor's action is a good example of what Richard Adelman (1995) has called in another context 'The Alzheimerization of Ageing'.

Old age, as Riordan and Whitmore (1990) note in their book, *Living with Dementia*, 'is an idea that arises out of culture not biology'. Given that our understanding often comes from medical explanations and media representations, most people will almost certainly have a negative view of Alzheimer's disease. The effect is that Alzheimer's disease becomes a medical issue and the individual a 'sufferer'. Whilst no one would want to suggest that the loss of previously taken-for-granted abilities is something to celebrate, most discussions about Alzheimer's involve negative assessments. Carers are viewed either as surrogate professional carers or as superhuman. The fact that they are in reality fulfilling a role based on love and/or friendship tends to be forgotten or ignored. There is little doubt that media representations tend to rely either on the dominant medical views of Alzheimer's, or on exposés examining poor treatment facilities. Yet the media is uncertain, as is our society generally, in its response towards the elderly who are often represented in terms of extremes. On the one hand there is peddled a line about the wisdom of age, on the other is a media obsessed with youth and rejuvenation. Moreover, all of this is often played against a backdrop of debates about the 'functionality' of those who have lived too long and issues about 'quality of life' and rights to existence. Such debates about the role of the elderly are easily transported into any discussion of Alzheimer's disease and it is unlikely that Alzheimer's disease, even if de-medicalised, would escape negative media representations altogether. Alzheimer's disease needs to be presented realistically, which means recognising that whilst individuals do change, this does not always equate with absolute negativity. Bayley (1998), for instance, found that Alzheimer's disease moved his relationship with his wife forward:

Every day, we move closer and closer together. We could not do otherwise. Purposefully, persistently, involuntarily, our marriage is now getting somewhere. It is giving us no choice, and I am glad of that. Every day, we are physically closer; and Iris's little 'mouse cry', as I think of it, signifying loneliness in the next room, the wish to be back beside me, seems less and less forlorn, more simple, more natural.

(Bayley, 1998)

Responsibility to others

The way we respond to each other depends on three factors: what we ourselves understand to be happening; the meaning we attach to that understanding and the conditions that allow us to act. Clearly, the last factor is dependent upon individual circumstances although, as we have already seen, there are probably a number of shared features of Alzheimer's disease that restrict an individual's ability to respond (Levin *et al*, 1989).

When we learn that somebody close to us has Alzheimer's disease, what happens? As indicated in an earlier chapter, we are likely to go through a process of bereavement; a process which may not, because of the duration of the illness, be satisfactorily resolved for a number of years, a fact aptly summed up in the title of Forsythe's (1990) book, *Alzheimer's Disease: the long bereavement.* Although this chapter is not primarily concerned with the debate about whether Alzheimer's is a straightforward disease or a response by society to certain behaviours (see, for example, Harding and Palfrey, 1997) one's own response to this question is important, for the question of the inevitability of deterioration unavoidably follows on. From a medical view it is known that a small number of dementing illnesses (about ten per cent) are reversible. We also know that the rest, particularly Alzheimer's, follow a fairly predictable course across all of those with the disease.

This clearly allows for great individual variation, a case in point being David Snowdon's (1997) contested study of Sister Mary, who lived until 101 years of age with high cognitive test scores, despite evidence of having Alzheimer's disease. Even though there are a great number of pharmacological and non-pharmacological approaches to Alzheimer's disease, there still appears to be, in the public mind at least, an assumption that nothing can be done, yet as Post (1995) notes, 'solidarity, comfort and reassurance are not nothing'.

Following on from what we understand to be happening, is the question of what it means to us. Alzheimer's disease throws up questions about personal identity in ways that many other illnesses do not. This is partly to do with the longevity of the mind-losing process — 'the maze of Alzheimer's disease' — and partly it is to do with the normal life that preceded it; a period of lucidity that no one knew would be interrupted. It also has to do with the question of whether Alzheimer's disease is an inevitable feature of ageing. The most important question, perhaps, is whether one can realistically still talk about the same person when all of their practical competencies and emotional responses have changed. Is the 'self' still the same? Is self-identity intact? These are questions that, when answered, have profound consequences since much of moral theory requires a self that can be known. In Alzheimer's disease such an ability to know oneself appears to be precisely the sphere that has been damaged. Post (1995) notes one solution to this:

> *Rather than allowing declining mental capacities to divide humanity into those who are worthy or unworthy of full moral attention, it is better to develop an ethics based on the essential unity of human beings and on an assertion of equality despite unlikeness of mind... I further think that full self-identity, made possible by an intact memory that connects past and present, should not be overvalued lest those who are disconnected from their pasts by forgetfulness be excluded from the protective canopy of 'do no harm'.*

(Post, 1995)

One result of seeing the person with memory loss as deprived of selfhood is to begin to relate to them in a different way. Martin Buber, the Jewish theologian, wrote in an influential book entitled, *I and Thou* (1970) that:

> *The life of a human being does not exist merely in the sphere of goal-directed verbs. It does not consist merely of activities that have something for their object. I perceive something. I feel something. I imagine something. I want something. I sense something. I think something. The life of a human being does not consist merely of all this and its like.*
>
> *All this and its like is the basis of the realm of the It.*
>
> *But the realm of You has another basis.*

(Buber, 1970)

Buber is making clear that we should not use other people as ends or means and that real relationships involve an openness to the other person. When we see other people as objects we enter into an I-It relationship. Some writers have suggested that an I-Thou relationship is beyond the normal scope of many people and that a more realistic relationship to be hoped for is I-You (Cox, 1965). Whether we accept this or not, the fundamental distinction is between a relationship based on treating the other as a person irrespective of what has happened to their cognitive abilities, and relating to them as a person where such faculties remain undisturbed and presumably undiminished. One is reminded here of Kierkegaard (1989) who noted that: 'The biggest danger, that of losing oneself, can pass off in the world as quietly as if it were nothing; every other loss, an arm, a leg, five dollars, a wife, etc. is bound to be noticed.' It does seem, in some of the more philosophical debates about Alzheimer's, that cognitive abilities make the person and that as long as these remain uncorrupted, the self which we all believe we have, marches on through life without obstruction.

Linda Grant (1998), in a recent account of her mother's mental deterioration, noted that 'Cancer is cancer, but when you lose your memory the whole family goes down with it and you must do what you can to reclaim yourselves from oblivion.' This is an important point and we need to remember that responsibility towards others is built on an acknowledgement of ourselves. Erich Fromm (1957), in *The Art of Loving*, notes that 'The affirmation of one's own life, happiness, growth, freedom is rooted in one's capacity to love, that is in care, respect, responsibility and knowledge. If an individual is able to love productively, he loves himself too; if he can only love others, he cannot love at all.' This is not simply a question of being strong so that we can cope with others, it is a fundamental point about the possibility of love. The I in the I-Thou relationship is not acting through moral duty, indeed the 'I' is not acting at all, but being. Bayley (1998) aptly sums up the dependence that is forged in the face of Alzheimer's disease when he states, 'The voyage is over and under the dark escort of Alzheimer's, she has arrived somewhere, so have I.'

Conclusion

TS Eliot, in 'Choruses from "The Rock"' (1964), asks, 'Where is the Life we have lost in living?'. This chapter has attempted to go some way to explore this question. It has not provided any of the answers since, as Victor Frankl noted (1959), 'meaning must be found, but cannot be given'. Instead, some of the ways in which we talk about Alzheimer's disease have been examined. Whilst this 'talk' is of vital and practical importance it does not (nor does it attempt to) answer or explore some of the more urgent questions arising in the minds of those who care for someone with Alzheimer's disease. Technical descriptions of the disease, however important, do not lead to greater self-understanding. Whilst it is a challenge for services to respond creatively to the needs of carers, there is arguably a greater challenge; namely to engage in dialogue about what Alzheimer's disease means to them. Currently medical discourse focuses on the individual brain pathology of Alzheimer's, and other health professionals focus on the behavioural problems associated with the disease. Talking to carers about what it means to have Alzheimer's is the next step, for as Wittgenstein (1961) reminds us, 'even when all possible scientific questions have been answered, the problems of life remain completely untouched'.

References

Adelman R (1995) The Alzheimerization of Ageing. *Gerontol* **35**(4): 526–32

Bauman Z (1992) *Mortality, Immortality & Other Life Strategies.* Polity Press, Cambridge

Bayley J (1998) 'Elegy for Iris'. The New Yorker, 27 July

de Beauvoir S (1972) *Old Age.* Penguin, Harmondsworth

Bonhoeffer D (1959) *Letters and Papers from Prison.* Fontana, London

Buber M (1970) *I and Thou.* T & T Clark, Edinburgh

Burns A, Howard R, Pettit W (1995) *Alzheimer's Disease: a medical companion.* Blackwell Science, Oxford

Cotrell V, Schulz R (1993) The perspective of the patient with Alzheimer's disease: A neglected dimension of dementia research. *Gerontol* **33**(2):205–11

Cox H (1965) *The Secular City.* Springer, New York

Davis R (1989) *My Journey ino Alzheimer's Disease.* Scripture Press, Amersham

Doerberg M (1989) *Stolen Mind: the slow disappearance of Ray Doerberg.* Algonquin, Chapel Hill, North Carolina

Eliot TS (1964) Choruses from 'The Rock'. *TS Eliot. Selected Poems.* Faber & Faber Ltd, London

Erikson E (1968) *Identity: Youth and Crisis.* Penguin, Harmondsworth

Forsythe E (1990) *Alzheimer's Disease: the long bereavement.* Faber & Faber, London

Frankl VE (1959) *Man's Search for Meaning.* Washington Square Press, New York

Fromm E (1957) *The Art of Loving.* Unwin Books, London

Gelder M, Gath D, Mayou R *et al* (1996) *Oxford Textbook of Psychiatry.* Oxford Univertity Press, Oxford

Goldsmith M (1996) *Hearing the Voice of People with Dementia: opportunities and obstacles.* Jessica Kingsley Publishing, London

Grant L (1998) *Remind Me Who I Am Again.* Granta, London

Harding N, Palfrey C (1997) *The Social Construction of Dementia: Confused Professionals.* Jessica Kingsley Publishing, London

Hoening J (1968) The de-segregation of the psychiatrist patient. *Proceedings of the Royal Society of Medicine* **61**: 115–20

Hoening J, Hamilton MW (1967) The burden on the household in an extramural psychiatric service. In: Freeman, Farndale, eds. *New Aspects of the Mental Health Services.* Pergamon, London

Kierkegaard S (1989) *The Sickness unto Death.* Penguin, Harmondsworth

Kitwood T, Bredin K (1992) Towards a theory of dementia care: person-hood and wellbeing. *Ageing and Society* 12: 269–87

Kushner HS (1981) *Bad Things Happen to Good People.* Shocken, New York

Levin E (1991) Carers – Problems, strains and services. In: Jacoby, Oppenheimer, eds. *Psychiatry in the Elderly.* Oxford University Press, Oxford

Levin E, Sinclair I, Gorbach P (1989) *Families, Services and Confusion in Old Age.* Gower, Aldershot

Mace NL, Rabins PV, Castleton BA *et al* (1988) *The 36-Hour Day: A family guide to caring at home for people with Alzheimer's disease and other confusional illnesses.* Age Concern, London

McGowin DF (1993) *Living in the Labyrinth: a personal journey through the maze of Alzheimer's.* Elder Books, San Fransisco

Platt S (1985) Measuring the Burden of psychiatric illness on the family: an evaluation of some rating scales. *Psychol Med* **15**: 383–93

Post SG (1995) *The Moral Challenge of Alzheimer's Disease.* John Hopkins University Press, Baltimore

Riordan J, Whitmore B (1990) *Living with Dementia.* Manchester University Press, Manchester

Schrum D (1989) To Reconsider One's Life: An exploration in meaning. In Paavo Pylkkanen, ed. *The Search for Meaning: The new spirit in science and philosophy.* Crucible, Wellingborough

Sinason V (1992) *Mental Handicap amd the Human Condition: New approaches from the Tavistock.* Free Associations Press, London

Snowdon DA (1997) Ageing and Alzheimer's Disease: Lessons from the Nun Study. *Gerontol* **37**(2): 150–6

Taylor R (1987) The Meaning of Life. In: Oswald Hanfling, ed. *Life and Meaning: A Reader.* Basil Blackwell, Oxford

Wittgenstein L (1961) *Tractatus Logico-Philosophicus.* Routledge & Kegan Paul, London

3

The eighth age of man: sociological reflections on Alzheimer's disease

David T Evans

> *... the fact that Alzheimer's is being recognised increasingly earlier — although... there is still no absolutely reliable diagnostic test — means that more people are having to face up to a positive diagnosis while they are still capable of understanding it.*
>
> (Hodgkinson, 1996: 51)

Introduction: The body

Until relatively recently, sociology has ignored what is perhaps the most obvious characteristic of human beings: we have bodies. It has also thereby suppressed an equally obvious 'fact' about human beings; namely that our bodies are not simply biological entities but are socially constructed through language, social interaction, visual representations and by communal practices (Turner, 1996).

In modern industrial societies, analyses of the human condition have been dominated by the basic opposition between the force of nature and the refining power of human culture, familiarly summarised as 'body versus mind' and 'body versus the soul', in which the superiority of culture over the raw material of nature — of mind and soul over body — has been assumed to be a necessary requirement for a truly civilised society. Descartes (1934) described the human body as a machine directed by instructions from the mind; only human reasoning can make sense of and give meaning to our experience of our own and others' bodies. Without our ability to reason and to develop rational explanations we would be without human culture, that quality which marks us apart from all other animals; we wouldn't exist as (thinking) human beings. As a consequence of this emphasis on the civilising triumph of mind over matter, philosophers and social scientists have been preoccupied with matters mental, cultural and spiritual, leaving the study of the human body and its workings to 'pure' sciences such as biology, physiology and genetics. However, whilst our bodies are undoubtedly physiological 'machines' which demand and require the attentions of 'pure' science, it is only through our choice and use of language, art, photography and sculpture that we are able to make any sense of them; to explain and describe issues of pain, health, fitness, illness, development and decline. Far from being merely physiological machines, human bodies are indeed the focus of a wealth of social descriptions, assumptions, feelings and value judgements, and as sociology constantly reminds us, the 'pure' sciences themselves can only develop and operate through the use of (elaborate, technical) language and imagery, within social organisations. These are governed by all manner of political and economic interests which affect and direct research, analysis and, where deemed appropriate, medical treatment and care. Medical research and practice rest as much with administrators and accountants (who also take decisions on what to research and treat and how) as with doctors and researchers. Thus, all aspects of medical maintenance and treatment are expressed and communicated through language, much of it generalised everyday descriptive language and euphemism, even slang, as well as the technical terminology of medical practice. In brief, 'pure' sciences are not pure in the literal sense of being outside social and cultural influence, but are themselves determined by social and political interests, values and decision-making.

Bodies and their attributes are not the sole preserve of medical practitioners and the patients they treat. As in all cultures whatever their stage of development, in societies such as our own, the body is the focus of widespread religious, folk and popular beliefs and preoccupations. Bodies are 'occupied' or 'owned' by individuals who constantly reflect upon and judge their shape, size, blemishes and pains. In the consumerist economies and cultures of North America, Australasia and Western Europe, there is a high premium on the cosmetically attractive, fit, 'worked-out', healthy-dieted and expensively-clothed body, judged by idealised standards of skin tone, breast and thigh shapes, stomach musculature and bottom firmness, and so on.

Within popular culture the 'heart' is not merely a critical body part, but an elaborately mystified component of our emotional and love lives. Our hearts have 'desires', we 'lose' our hearts, 'break' them, and so on. Nor is the 'mind', supposedly the driver of this bodily machine, simply dependent upon the functioning of neural matter, but the means by which we interpret ideas, solve tasks and process feelings and emotions into thoughts and words. We believe that our minds reflect our personalities and if we 'lose' our minds we lose our sanity and thereby our coherent identity. We comment on people being 'quick-' or 'slow-witted' and praise those who have 'lively' and 'fascinating' minds and/or 'great' personalities. We are somewhat in awe of those who are 'clever' or 'brainy'. By contrast, we make little sense of those who have apparently lost their reason.

Overall, our obsessions with having and maintaining 'youthful' bodies and lifestyles, synonymously imply having alert, active and lively minds. Clearly the body is not merely a physical/genetic entity, but a complex social construction. Indeed, with current scientific progress in genetics and transsexual surgery, the human body is arguably destined to be, in the not too distant future, not *even* a physical/genetic entity.

On the whole, ageing and death are denied and ignored within this scenario of cosmetic renewal and 'youthfulness', but beneath these surface preoccupations we have a rapidly ageing or 'greying' population for whom the mental and bodily ravages of disease, illness and disability become increasingly threatening and costly.

Within the boundaries of modern reasoning, illness and disease are due to a disturbance in the symbiotic relationship between body and mind. Indeed, the very word 'disease' originates in the French *desaise*, indicating an impairment of ease or comfort; the splitting of body and mind, the mind's loss of control over the body. In the modern era there has been strict regulation of the emotions and close disciplining of a body perceived as potentially dangerous; as a possible channel for the unruly, raw and destructive forces of nature (Foucault 1973, 1979), 'disease' thus signifying a partial or complete loss of cultural control over nature. The scientific battle to assert and strengthen the rightful rule of reason over nature has been developed and monitored by various professional institutions including the medical, but also effectively rests on the prime need in a civilised world to instil in us all the virtues of self-regulation if we are to qualify as truly moral subjects. In medical terms, we are expected to be able to identify symptoms of any breakdown in this regulation and maintenance of the body; to detect signs of illness and disease in relatives and friends. The implications for us as individuals living with our own bodies have been described as living with bodies which over time, as we experience their changing shapes, functioning and efficiency, become 'the inscribed surface of events'; which remind us that our bodies are 'in perpetual disintegration' (Foucault, 1979).

Age as a social category (like class, occupation, religion or ethnicity) is clearly socially constructed. Regardless of their personal differences, individuals can be located in age categories broadly characteristic of the key stages of life and referred to in traditional societies as 'the seven ages of man'. These stages may vary from society to society but in most, age confers wisdom, respect, valued experience and responsibility within the close-knit social context of extended family networks and community. In societies such as ours, these qualities are at least qualified and even challenged by the emphasis on youth, health and consumerism.

As with illness and disease, the notion that ageing is socially constructed does not require us to deny that it is also a biological process involving a decline in physical ability, the emergence of grey hair, a decline in skin texture, an increase in the brittleness of the skeletal structure and, eventually, a decline in mental ability. However, the social value, meaning and response to these biological processes can vary enormously and in a consumerist culture in which perpetual, even if cosmetically achieved, youthfulness, vitality and alertness are valued above all other qualities, the paradox of being able to 'live', or rather 'age' longer is uneasily met.

So human bodies, though existing of organic matter, only have meaning as a result of cultural communication and social interaction. Both may be exercised through the complexities of 'expert' scientific enquiry or through everyday interaction. Either way, bodies and their parts are clearly socially constructed. Rather than the body being a machine driven by the mind, the mind through its thoughts, ideas and reasoning 'constructs' the body, defines its shape and health and elaborates upon its defects and diseases.

Given the particular concerns of this text it is hoped that the reader will already have identified the affront that Alzheimer's disease and other dementias pose. Alzheimer's disease marks the splitting not only of mind from body, but also of fragments of the disintegrating mind from each other as the mind's power over the body is progressively eroded. It also marks our inability to understand the collapse of rationality, culminating in a condition which so many texts intended to be guides for carers, helpers and relatives, simply describe as 'mysterious' or 'the cruellest disease' (a relative of a sufferer quoted by Sweeting and Gilhooly, 1997). Alzheimer's disease is perhaps most succinctly and poignantly understood when placed alongside the first Cartesian principle of modern existence: 'I think therefore I am.'

The body has become important in contemporary culture as a consequence of major changes in the nature of medical practice and technology, and the changing structure of disease and illness in advanced industrial societies. The greying of populations has major sociological (ethical, philosophical, economic and legal) implications with regard to the issues of person-hood, consciousness, identity, individualism and so forth. The characteristics and prevalence of modern forms of degenerative disease are obviously closely related to the ageing of populations and the emergence of new 'killer diseases': diseases of the circulatory system, the respiratory system and malignant neoplasms (Turner, 1996), to which can be added the most 'mysterious' and frightening chronic illnesses of them all: the social and mental disintegration of Alzheimer's and other dementias.

Perhaps it would be useful, before turning our attention to sociological reflections on Alzheimer's disease, to illustrate sociological claims that bodies and bodily parts exist through language, symbolism and social values, by briefly referring to a telling example used by Turner in *The Body and Society* (1996); that of gout which is partly hereditary but also associated with poor diet, lack of exercise and alcoholism. As readers will no doubt be aware, the cause of gout is an accumulation of uric acid in the blood and the site of painful attack is normally the joint of the big toe. As Turner notes, this disease 'has all the features of an uncontrolled invasion of the body as a natural environment' (ibid.); the swollen and painful toe joints certainly may be analysed as objective 'thing-like' parts of the body, but gout has become socially inscribed in far more detail than this: 'Gout can also become part of the ensignia and stigmata of the personality, since part of the individuality of a person can be known from their gait' (ibid.).

Gout in the foot becomes a 'gouty personality' associated with an easy and rich lifestyle, and because of the effect on personal mobility it also becomes associated with leisureliness. Gout thus becomes associated with status; it is part of a total human identity. Indeed, almost all illnesses and diseases convey reflections of the personalities or identities of their 'owners' to the extent that ability to 'survive' through regimes of self-regulated, especially 'alternative', medical treatments for such chronic illnesses as those normally referred to as 'AIDS-related', is generally taken to be a sign of the 'strength' and 'fight' of the 'survivors', implying that a root cause of non-survival is some form of personality or identity weakness.

In these and other ways, disease is a cultural contradiction; it appears to be in nature and yet it is, at the same time and inevitably, deeply social. As Sontag (1983, 1988) has demonstrated in her works on cancer and later on AIDS, diseases carry metaphorical meanings which invariably implicate the patient's responsibility for their illness in some way, for failing in the constant human struggle of reason over nature. Similarly the metaphorical body is at the heart of all religious myths underpinned by parables of purity and danger (Douglas, 1966). In short:

> *The body offers a profound and rich source of metaphors and similes and modes of conceptualization for the crises, hazards, dangers and paradoxes of individual and collective existence.*
>
> (Turner, 1996)

The extent to which such metaphors and similes may be drawn from Alzheimer's disease, however, would appear to be very limited. Essentially they would appear to vary little from the basic images and signs of 'social death'.

The 'social death' of the demented body

> *We can without contradiction believe that dementia and Alzheimer's disease are medical categories which socially construct the problems of ageing into definite medical categories which allocate power to professional, social groups and believe that ageing is a real process taking place in the organic foundations of human embodiment.*
>
> (Turner, 1996)

Given the body/mind dualism and the superior value of the mind over the body within our cultural tradition, disintegration of the mind is the ultimate uncontrolled invasion of the body as a natural environment, and ultimately leaves the body 'lifeless', or as it is now more commonly expressed, 'socially dead': that is, its owner is perceived and/or treated as a 'non-person' for: 'socially he is already dead, though his body remains biologically alive' (Glaser and Strauss, 1966; see also Sudnow, 1967; Kastenbaum, 1972 and Kalish, 1968). Unfortunately for patients, carers, relatives and medical staff, perceptions and treatments of patients will rarely agree as to whether 'social death' has occurred: 'it is quite possible for an individual to be at the same time dead for some parties yet socially alive for others' (Mulkay, 1993).

Disease involves a loss of bodily, and in the case of Alzheimer's, mental ownership. It is the most extreme form of 'loss of self', not least because it is a 'self' also lost to relatives and friends. We remember first symptoms and fears as to their meanings, our first approach to GPs for their interpretations, subsequent developments, and so on. Such narratives (or personal accounts) appear to be especially important for the sufferers of chronic illnesses such as cancer and even other neurological disorders such as Parkinson's disease in which, whilst there is a slowing of reaction and thinking, memory is 'often relatively intact until the later stages in those whose intellect ultimately fails' (Wilcock, 1990).

With demographic changes and technical advances, the greying of populations has been accompanied by the increased cultural recognition of the split between biological and social deaths, and the need to define the 'loss of person-hood' (Sweeting and Gilhooly, 1997) indicated by the latter. Qualities of 'person-hood' include individual/personal power over life choices, the capacity for interpersonal relationships and interaction with others sharing the same culture, awareness or consciousness of the self as a social actor expressed in and through language and encompassing feelings and emotions about self pride, honour, satisfaction, and so on. However, 'In practice, the ability to recognise others appears to be the most important determinant of whether or not social death occurs' (ibid.). When the patient is a 'person' by these criteria, the medical process is one in which the voice of the patient is an important part, now commonly recognised as being 'heard' through patients' narratives. It is usually the 'owner', in interaction with relatives or close confidantes, who determines, possibly through a lengthy interpretative process, that there is something 'wrong'. But referral to a medical specialist does not end the patient's active role in the social construction of the disease's development or his/her career as a patient.

Given the extent to which experts' rational knowledge has been so highly valued in modern societies, it comes as no surprise that until the past two or so decades, doctors treated the personal accounts of their patients with scepticism given that they were outside the authority of the dominant biomedical voice:

> *The clinical gaze of the medical professions was focused on the inner bodily world of the patients. How patients spoke about their ills, symptoms and problems, was regarded as at best a pale reflection of the language of the organs and tissues and their pathological changes.*

(Hydén, 1997)

However, personal accounts are important in expressing our sense of self-image; how we perceive, experience and judge our lives (Ochberg, 1988) and how we assess what is happening in and to them, in short, 'how we make sense of the (our) social world' (Somers, 1994). Normally understood in terms of changes over time, dynamic events are linked to perceived changes in the identity or status of self as the narrator *negotiates*, in the case of chronic illnesses, with dramatically changed (disrupted) circumstances (Bury, 1982). The importance of narratives to medical practitioners is now recognised as crucial, but their importance to patients is mainly rooted in the way they serve as a mechanism for maintaining a sense of individual identity, of 'selfdom', through the clinical processes of becoming a diseased body, an illness, a prolonged death. Thus, amongst the chronically ill, it is well researched how AIDS and cancer patients constantly use narratives to re-negotiate their identities through the successive stages of their illnesses (Matheson and Stam, 1995).

We don't give accounts of our illnesses which are literally accurate and precise, rather we interpret them in ways which make sense to ourselves and possibly reinterpret them again when we describe them to key people such as doctors or nurses. From this point of view, our personal accounts of our illnesses as patients may vary depending upon the significance we give to them, who we are talking to and the possible consequences. We might suspect that a persistent pain has a 'serious' cause but may not refer to its persistence or painfulness when we first approach a doctor, yet we might well express our deepest fears to a close friend. In other words, our personal accounts of our illnesses vary according to who we are talking to and where we are talking to them. The ill and diseased do not produce a single narrative of their illnesses and diseases, but different narratives determined by situational factors, particularly the interaction between narrator and listener, patient and doctor, nurse, relative or carer (Clark and Mishler, 1992).

It is now a commonplace that becoming a patient, setting in motion the sequence of decision-making and interpretative processes, involves a series of negotiations and choices by the possible future patient from accepting that he or she is 'ill' to doing something about it (MacKinlay, 1973). The sequence of interactions which comes from suspecting and then accepting that one is 'ill', may later develop with the greater authoritative input of healthcare practitioners, but the patient remains their own key 'narrator' for the illness's development. These, often initially highly imprecise and vague patient accounts, instigate a socially defined illness or disease as something merely bodily 'wrong'. Dementias such as Alzheimer's, described in common-sense terms as 'mysterious' and represented as fateful random invasions of the body, are meticulously researched and analysed within medical science and remain the critical focus for elaborate narratives by the patient and all who interact with the patient throughout the stages of the disease's development.

Chronic illness creates a dependency on others and on medical technology, and patients' accounts also become dependent upon their interactions with carers, relatives, and especially the 'scripted' goals of the medical staff upon whom they depend. Accounts of the cultural context of hospice care demonstrate that for medical staff, the careful management of stress requires the development of a value system which regulates the meaning, importance and effects of the experience (Pearlin, 1989), as is clear from the following observation:

> *The resilience of those who choose and continue to work exclusively in this field is won by a full understanding of what is happening and not by a retreat behind a technique... if we are to remain for long near the suffering of dependence and parting we need also to develop a basic philosophy and search often painfully for meaning even in the most adverse situations.*

> (Saunders and Baines, 1983)

Such a basic philosophy is built around belief in an 'acceptable way of dying' (Aries, 1974), an 'appropriate death' (Blauner, 1966), a 'social death' (Mulkay, 1991) or, as those interviewed by McNamara *et al* (1995) referred to it, 'the good death' where there is 'awareness, acceptance and preparation' by the patient for death, arising out of a 'recounselling of dying people towards the acceptance of death' (McNamara *et al*, 1995). As one hospice nurse states, 'It is a good death when you feel you have contributed' (ibid.).

Patient accounts involving 'identity work' and nursing staff scripting towards 'the good death' outcome are both severely tested by Alzheimer's disease. It is characterised as the progressive 'disintegration' (or disembodiment) of the actor-patient at the centre, leaving other key actors: close relatives, friends, carers and medical staff, literally 'on stage' with leading actors who forget or say the wrong lines, don't recognise who they are talking to or know where the 'audience' is, get their costumes and make-up all wrong, and so on. Not surprisingly, for these other actors the effect can only be 'strange and frightening' (Forsythe, 1996). The critical cancer patient narratives referred to by Matheson and Stam (1995) are presumably denied to those suffering from Alzheimer's disease once past the 'early confusional phase' (Greutzner, 1997). However:

> ... *the fact that Alzheimer's is being recognised increasingly earlier — although... there is still no absolutely reliable diagnostic test — means that more people are having to face up to a positive diagnosis while they are still capable of understanding it.*

(Hodgkinson, 1996)

Inevitably, their facing up to such a positive diagnosis will initially be informed by media coverage which gives Alzheimer's a frightening and fearsome reputation. There are no cures or known causes; diagnostic confirmation rests on brain biopsies after death. All there is, is the grim inevitability of mental and social death before biological death. Indeed, — so mysterious and terrifying is Alzheimer's — in a greying population it threatens us all. In Britain there are currently approximately 600,000 sufferers of dementias, 55.6 per cent with Alzheimer's, and its incidence is 'likely to rise by 25 % in the next generation as people live longer' (Stuttaford, 1998).

> *The size of the problem (of dementia) is going to escalate rapidly, especially in the next twenty years. Of those aged sixty-five to seventy, it appears that approximately one person in twenty has dementia, but the proportion of sufferers rises with increasing age, and of those over the age of seventy-five, one person in five will probably have some degree of dementia. The number of older people in our population is expected to increase greatly between now and the early years of the next century, and by far the largest proportional increase will be in those seventy-five and over. The simplest of the medical definitions of dementia is 'a global loss of intellectual function that is usually progressive and in the majority but not all cases untreatable'.*

(Wilcock,1990)

The accounts of identity change through the disease's developmental stages may be denied the patient, but they are certainly not denied carers, friends or relatives. Indeed, the latter may well feel the need to act as surrogate narrators in order to somehow 'make sense' of the disease and to retain some sort of lasting coherent identity for the individual undergoing the disintegrative process.

Dr Elizabeth Forsyth notes, at the start of her quest to unravel the mysteries of Alzheimer's disease from which her husband, John, suffered and died, 'During my quest in the years since his death I have realised that nobody who dies from Alzheimer's disease could write the story of his own life without much outside help' (Forsythe, 1996). Her text is in major part intended as John's 'narrative', indeed six other similar second-hand Alzheimer 'narratives' are also provided by her, and as one might expect they represent more the narratives of carers than of patients. Hints as to how the 'identity' challenge of Alzheimer's *might* be reported by Alzheimer's sufferers, are provided in the narratives of those suffering from comparable, though less severe, mentally debilitating diseases.

Research into the personal accounts of sufferers from Parkinson's disease (Nijhof, 1995) demonstrate their keen sense of shame at early symptoms of the decline in their social and mental competence. In accounts such as provided by Forsythe (1996), it appears that with Alzheimer's disease, in the early stages especially, similar feelings are transposed onto relatives and other close carers. If sufferers of Alzheimer's are aware in the early stages that they are indeed sufferers, diagnostic accounts invariably record compensatory tendencies of denial, possibly induced through fear or confusion, or indeed, perhaps, shame-induced attempts to cover up or hide initial lapses of memory, concentration, or speech.

Nijhof (1995) opens his account of sufferers from Parkinson's disease, focusing on their shame in their public appearance, by graphically describing the dilemmas of the patient/narrator.

Nijhof's respondents talk in a litany including such words and phrases as 'shame', 'disgrace', 'terrible', 'horribly', 'hide signs of', 'not daring something', because there is a recognition that they will not act in accordance with accepted standards; expressions such as 'being noticed', 'being looked at', and so on, are frequently used. Nijhof identifies four sets of related rules of 'normal' competence (in standing, walking, eating, speaking, etc.) of which his respondents were aware, or feared breaking. They perceived such lapses in terms of falling short of adult competence, that is of their being childlike in carrying out the most ordinary and mundane everyday life actions which are normally merely taken for granted and not referred to explicitly, but which reflect on such basic, highly-valued human qualities as independence, competence and decency.

The reference to being 'childlike' is especially revealing. As Wilcock (1990) states of the later stages of Alzheimer's disease where there is total dependence:

> *The physical side of the illness becomes more apparent and it is easier for most people to relate to this. In many instances they have looked after a physically dependent person, such as a young child, in the past, and caring for a person with dementia in this final phase is in many ways similar to looking after a child. The sad thing is of course that in the case of a child, one anticipates that the problem will diminish as the child grows older, whereas in the case of someone with dementia, it is going to get worse.*

> (Wilcock, 1990)

Critically, 'public exposure' causes the greatest embarrassment, forcing relatives and patients to feel it necessary to 'hide early signs' by removing the self or patient from the 'public domain'. There is a 'splitting of the life-world' (Giddens, 1991) between public shame and the private sphere where 'symptoms lose their shamefulness'. Like Parkinson's disease, Alzheimer's disease is in this sense, for relatives and friends if not for the sufferers themselves, a 'located disease', and as the retreat from 'shame' accelerates, the location moves inexorably into confinement. However, this does not necessarily mean institutionalised confinement — far from it:

> *Most studies (show that) only 15 – 20% or less of people with dementia are living permanently in an institution, and that a large proportion of those that are, are living in old people's homes, rather than geriatric hospitals.*

> (Wilcock, 1990)

Sweeting and Gilhooly's (1997) analysis of the perceptions and emotional reactions of relatives of dementia sufferers is based on questionnaire responses rather than personal accounts as such, though their findings suggest patterned accounts of their experiences which might well be expressed in narrative form. These were relatives of sufferers diagnosed with primary senile dementia who were therefore well past the early stage of 'public shaming' referred to above. Even so, the majority (about 60 per cent), though believing the sufferers to be in some sense 'socially dead', nevertheless continued to behave as if the sufferers were socially alive. The authors identify four categories of relative narratives:

1   ***Believing and behaving as though the sufferer was socially dead:*** *'... really the person has died and you're just left with the body, that's how I feel about her...'; '... we treat her mostly, unfortunately, as if she's not really in our world'; 'death would come as a blessing'; 'They become a different person really'; 'it's like living with the living dead'.*

2   ***Believing the sufferer was socially dead but behaving as if they were still alive, even though still thinking that the sufferer's death would be a blessing:*** *'I think if they're just left to sit in a chair they just vegetate – just lose interest, do nothing, you know'; 'You know he's all involved he's still there'.*

3   ***Behaving as though the sufferer was socially dead without believing that they were.*** *This was a very rare scenario but was typified by discounting the sufferer's social presence whilst maintaining that the latter's quality of life was sufficient (for example, by seeming happy and being physically fit) to claim that death would not be a blessing.*

4   ***Neither believing nor behaving as though the sufferer was socially dead:*** *'Make a joke of it, don't say "that's stupid" – don't make it obvious they can't do a thing... You don't embarrass them by having to cut food for them – have it cut before you put it on their plate – but not too small, let them work away a wee bit themselves...'; '... he said "Hello" and that meant he knew me...'.*

The narratives of relatives and carers of sufferers from Alzheimer's have not only to make sense of a disease which at present defeats 'pure' medical science, they also have to, somehow, through their retrospective accounts, hold on to the 'person-hood', the identity of the person socially dying before them. Forsythe (1996) records, 'I have heard Alzheimer's disease called "a slow goodbye" or an "ongoing bereavement" or the "empty house syndrome".' These all describe the long-lasting pain of watching someone you *once* knew change and disintegrate in this growing 'eighth age of man' in a culture which overtly celebrates, commercially sells and idealises the fit, beautiful, ageless body and ever-youthful mind. With an ever-increasing number living into their seventies, eighties and nineties, there will be a proportional increase in the numbers who will pass through 'social death' before they biologically pass away.

Whilst Alzheimer's disease is a progressive, disintegrative, neural disease manifested through a gradual memory decline, emotional response, language skills and mobility, its full meaning is built out of cultural communication and social interaction, interpreted through media coverage, 'expert' research, healthcare practices, the everyday interactions of all key actors and their narratives. Alzheimer's may apparently represent the ultimate defeat of culture and reason by invasive nature, but also it may only be identified, addressed and comprehended, as a socially constructed condition.

Note

Greutzner (1997) distinguishes between five diagnostic stages in the development of Alzheimer's disease whilst other writers identify different numbers of stages, but all recognise the arbitrariness of such a diagnostic guide. For Greutzner, the Early Confusional Stage 1 (forgetfulness becomes a problem, and confusion and slower responses affect such activities as driving; some problems with social conversation emerge; there are some detectable signs of personality changes, and so on, all possibly subject to claims of denial by the person concerned) is followed successively by those escalating symptoms organised under the headings of Late Confusional Stage 2, through Early Dementia Stage 3 and Middle Dementia Stage 4, to Late Dementia Stage 5.

In contrast, Wilcock (1990) identifies 'roughly' three stages, defined to a greater extent by the reactions of significant others (relatives, friends, and so on), in the first stage of which behavioural symptoms may be those generally (and incorrectly) associated with ageing, but which may be symptomatic of a number of dementias. The second stage is one in which the 'deterioration in ability makes it clear to everyone that something is wrong, and that it is no longer a question, even stretching the imagination considerably, that normal ageing is still the problem.' The third stage is one of total dependence.

References

Aries P (1974) *Western Attitudes Towards Death*. John Hopkins University Press, Baltimore

Blauner R (1966) Death and social structure. *Psychiatry* **29**: 378–94

Bury M (1982) Chronic illness as biographical disruption. *Sociol Health Ill* **4**: 167–82

Clark JA, Mishler EG (1992) Attending patients' stories: reframing the clinical task. *Sociol Health Ill* **14**: 344–71

Descartes R (1934) *Discourse on Method*. J M Dent and Son, New York

Douglas M (1966) *Purity and Danger: An Analysis of Concepts of Pollution and Taboo*. Penguin, Harmondsworth

Forsythe E (1996) *The Mystery of Alzheimer's: A Guide for Carers*. Kyle Cathie Ltd, London

Foucault M (1973) *The Birth of the Clinic: An Archaeology of Medical Perception*. Penguin, Harmondsowrth

Foucault M (1979) *Discipline and Punish: The Birth of the Prison*. Penguin, Harmondsworth

Giddens A (1991) *Modernity and Self-Identity: Self and Society in the Late Modern Age*. Cambridge University Press, Cambridge

Glaser BG, Strauss AL (1966) *Awareness of Dying*. Aldine Press, Chicago

Greutzner H (1997) *Alzheimer's: The Complete Guide for Families and Loved Ones: A Caregiver's Guide and Sourcebook*. John Wiley and Sons, New York

Hodgkinson L (1996) *Alzheimer's Disease: Your Questions Answered*. Ward Lock, London

Hydén LC (1997) Illness and narrative. *Sociol Health Ill* **19**(1):48–69

Kalish RA (1968) Life and death – dividing the invisible. *Soc Sci Med* **2**: 249–59

Kastenbaum RJ (1972) While the old man dies: our conflicting attitudes towards the elderly. In: Schoenberg B, Carr AC, Peretz D *et al* eds. *Psychological Aspects of Terminal Care*. Columbia University Press, New York

Matheson CM, Stam HJ (1995) Renegotiating identity: cancer narratives. *Sociol Health Ill* **17**(3): 283–306

McKinlay JB (1973) Social Networks, lay consultation and help-seeking behaviour. *Social Faces* **51**: 255–92

McNamara B, Waddell C, Colvin M (1995) Threats to the good death: the cultural context of stress among hospice nurses. *Sociol Health Ill* **17**(2): 222–6

Mulkay M (1991) The changing profile of social death. *Arch Européennes de Sociologie* **32**:172–96

Mulkay M (1993) Social death in Britain. In: Clark D ed. *The Sociology of Death: Theory, Culture, Practice*. Blackwell, Oxford

Nijhof G (1995) Parkinson's disease as a problem of shame in public appearance. *Sociol Health Ill* **17**:(2): 193–205

Ochberg RL (1988) Life stories and the psychosocial construction of careers. *J Pers* **56**: 173–204

Pearlin L (1989) The sociological study of stress. *J Health Soc Behav* **30**: 241–56

Saunders C, Baines M (1983) *Living with Dying: The Management of Terminal Disease*. Oxford University Press, Oxford

Somers MR (1994) The narrative constitution of identity: a relational and network approach. *Theory and Society* **23**: 605–49

Sontag S (1983) *Illness as Metaphor*. Penguin, London

Sontag S (1988) *AIDS and its Metaphors*. Penguin, London

Stuttaford T (1998) 'New drug to ease signs of dementia'. The Times, 28 May: 20

Sudnow D (1967) *Passing On: The Social Organisation of Dying*. Prentice-Hall Inc., Englewood Cliffs

Sweeting H, Gilhooly M (1997) Dementia and the phenomenon of social death. *Sociol Health Ill* **19**(1): 93–117

Turner BS (1996) *The Body and Society,* 2nd edn. Sage, London

Wilcock G (1990) *Living with Alzheimer's Disease and Similar Conditions*. Penguin, Harmondsworth

Part 2:
Psychological and practical aspects of care

4

Love, loss, and disappearing lives

Matthew V Morrissey

*Central to the devastating effects of Alzheimer's disease for
the carer, are the relentless demands of care and the cruel,
steady, crippling loss of the person.*

(Matthew V Morrissey, 1999)

This chapter will examine loss and bereavement in relation to carers,
families and Alzheimer's disease. It will be shown that honesty, love
and compassion are key ingredients in aiding the process of care. Such
qualities are born out of an implicit trust in and desire to be with people
who are suffering with or affected by Alzheimer's disease. It is also clear
from research on carers' perspectives that practical skills, information,
education, and counselling are not enough (Heyman, 1995; Morrissey,
1997). What is more important is to develop the spiritual, emotional and
psychological aspects of care and support. It is hoped that this brief
discussion will offer some understanding of loss and bereavement in the
everyday lives of carers and offer some suggestions to help support all
those involved in care including children.

Caring and loss of self

Carl Rogers is one of several humanistic psychologists who have
helped us to understand our 'self' (Rogers, 1984). Equally, however,
social psychologists such as Elliot Aronson help us to understand the
complex nature of our emotional lives (Aronson, 1988), for example,
the fact that we may take it for granted that a person we love will
always be there. Such predictability is part of what we need to form
close emotional bonds and human relationships.

Unpredictable events can cause great loss, hurt and pain — if, for
example, a member of our family should die suddenly. However, it seems
equally difficult and even more puzzling for family and relatives to come
to terms with the gradual and sometimes sudden loss of 'self' of the person
they knew before the onset of Alzheimer's disease. It is true to say that the
person is disappearing and, frighteningly, in some cases is already gone.

Central to the devastating effects of Alzheimer's disease for the carer, are the relentless demands of care and the cruel, steady, crippling loss of the person. So at the same time that a carer is having to come to terms with the burden of care-giving, they are required to respond in the right way and come to terms with their own feelings of loss. The closer the bond and the knowledge of the person, the more noticeable the losses.

Many individuals are aware that they are losing their mental functions and many try to cover up. However, the first stages of loss may go undetected by both the person with Alzheimer's and their family. The main reason for this is that diagnosis may take time and the condition is often undetected. When a diagnosis is absent, carers try to grapple with difficulties in great confusion, with little or no support. Such attempts often mean that carers themselves become ill under the ever-increasing burden of care (Warner, 1995).

> *I always worry leaving her. I know the nurses are very good but I have been looking after her for years more or less on my own. I cry sometimes on my way home as she just isn't my wife any more. I come here during the day sometimes as I only sit and worry at home and the staff don't mind.*

(Carer)

> *People with dementia go through a period of depression when they realise what's happening, and that's a terrible thing to watch, at one stage I thought it cruel to keep her alive.*

(Josceline Dimbleby, cited in Pickles, 1998)

Moira is a sixty-eight years old married lady and has four grown-up children and seven grandchildren. She comes from a close-knit and loving family. Recently she was diagnosed with Alzheimer's disease. She admits that she feels very depressed and is aware of her mental deterioration. She feels terrified for the future and has already started attending a day centre.

Sadly, Moira is one of millions of people world wide whose life is disappearing as the onset and ravages of Alzheimer's disease take over. Loss is a very real experience for the individual and their family on a level indescribable and unimaginable to people who have no direct experience of care. Providing support for individuals and their family is important at this early stage, and there is a real need to develop support groups (Yale, 1995).

From the outset, the topic of loss and Alzheimer's disease touches on almost everything related to being a person, including the robbing of dignity, independence and individuality. More importantly, families in the nineties face a huge crisis given recent changes in traditional family life. In the past, when the extended family was the norm, a 'caring network' was always in place (Iverson, 1988). However, divorce, job mobility and the two-breadwinner family has destroyed that safety net. In the nineties, many individuals have to juggle the conflicting demands of children, ageing parents, career and partner (Pickles, 1998).

Many carers are aware of the struggle in trying to achieve the best care for their relatives, given competing demands and often poor education, practical support and/or resources. Yet on top of the burden of care, carers are expected, often unaided, to learn about Alzheimer's disease and also to come to terms with the enormity of their own experiences of loss (Kreiner, 1995).

Clearly, taking on the role of a primary carer can sometimes create an intense and continuous conflict area for families. These types of conflict have recently been described by Linda Grant, a novelist and journalist. Her book documents the pain and the dilemma that she faced and which led to the decision to put her elderly mother with dementia in a nursing home (Grant, 1998). The book documents, in many ways, the awful feelings of loss and conflict that arise when a parent develops dementia.

Linda Grant recognises that, although times have changed, the dilemma of how to cope with ageing relatives and especially those with dementia remains. Clearly not all relationships between parents and their children are straightforward or harmonious. Sometimes the demands of care ignite sibling rivalry in establishing the boundaries and provision of care. This conflict within families may reflect previous conflict which is exacerbated by the demands of care. Additionally, trying to find support is difficult enough for professional people, but can be impossible for impoverished families. Little support from the state (Warner, 1995; Morrissey and Hill, 1997) means having either no support at all, or very few options for some families.

Once care is established, the views of the primary carer may not be taken seriously by professionals and this often results in confusion or a battle for access to basic and specialist services. The plight of carers in relation to this is well documented (Hicks, 1988; Mace and Rabins, 1991; Yale 1995; Morrissey and Hill, 1997). Such experiences can lead to disempowerment and a real feeling of loss of control, experienced first in relation to organising care and support, and later as the result of caring and/or death (Jones and Martinson, 1992). It is not surprising that, with such a burden of care, many carers fail to access support for themselves.

There lies a vulnerability between professional services and carers; a rending vulnerability felt when one partner goes into full-time care. The elderly partner who is able to live independently is often alone. Many carers travel long distances to visit their partners and relatives, and the devotion many have is incredible in spite of their own ill health and frailty.

> *I pace the house all night sometimes, I worry about her, it's silly really but I have cared for her all these years and I know she isn't coming back.*

> (Carer)

Alzheimer's is difficult emotionally for those professional carers who recognise the gaps in care.

> *I often sit there for a while, and really you can feel how lonely these families are caring for their mother, but it is not my job and I'm not sure whose job it is.*

> (Community psychiatric nurse)

In practice, the personal aspects of care must go hand in hand with education, counselling and support. More importantly the spiritual dimension of care is often unaddressed by medicine (Dyson, 1997). Care, therefore, could be viewed as a form of love, given that health professionals promise a consistent, skilled and informed concern, including a respect for individual dignity and rights. It has been suggested that we see professional care as a form of 'moderated love' (Campbell, 1984). However, with the experience of love comes the experience of loss.

The experiences of love and loss are clearly bound up in the fabric of our relationships, however superficial. Also, we become attached to aspects of our friends of which we are never aware until they leave or we are separated. There is a comfort in knowing that we are loved even though, sadly, many people find such feelings as hard to express as they do the feelings of loss. What is clear from my experience as a nurse and carer is that individuals have their own way of describing their emotional life. We need to listen to carers and families in a way that is not bound up by competing theories and personal philosophies. As a nurse one can be intelligent without being distant. One can learn much from what I call 'living knowledge', that is, the knowledge of doing and caring. Indeed, the main aspects of support depend to a large extent on our empathetic understanding of attachment and human relationships.

Attachment

Attachments and attachment figures are important to the stability of our emotional lives. In much of the theory surrounding attachment, the main focus has been to confirm that forming such emotional bonds is to maintain stability in life (Bowlby, 1980). However, in the case of Alzheimer's disease such attachment can lead to instability, as the carer may start to grieve before the person dies. The experience is emotionally complicated for the carer as the person they are caring for is still alive and continuing to require care. This is often compounded by feelings of guilt and a wall of fears surrounding loss, separation and eventually death. It is interesting to note that although attachment theory helps us to explore why and how attachments are formed, it cannot predict individual reactions.

Perhaps the nature of Alzheimer's disease forces us to address not only our attachments or lack of them, but also the nature of the attachments, which may indeed be equally painful. Traditionally, bereavement has been associated with loss through death of someone to whom there has been a strong emotional or loving attachment. Clearly, issues surrounding loss and Alzheimer's disease are not so clear cut. It is evident that much of the bereavement is experienced while the person is still alive (Jones and Martinson, 1992).

Reactions to Alzheimer's disease

The symptoms of Alzheimer's disease in the sufferer are sometimes mirrored in the reactions of carers to the ravages of the disease on their loved ones. For example, feelings of helplessness, crying, fear of loss, searching for meaning, searching for what to do, losing and finding parts of the old relationship, being afraid to leave the person, clinging to any form of hope and, sometimes, loss and grief reactions. Significant loss can also be experienced when a person moves from their familiar home surroundings to an institutional setting, however comfortable.

The sad fact is that all these types of loss, and still more, are experienced by both carers and those who suffer from Alzheimer's disease. Clearly, wrong assumptions can easily be made about the significance and intensity of attachments and this then results in inappropriate, uncaring responses.

Arrogant assumptions are sometimes fuelled under the surface by ageist attitudes which can sometimes result in elder abuse (Ogg and Bennett, 1992). Ageist attitudes are sometimes reflected in subtle ways, for example the belief that old peoples' relationships don't matter or are less important. Clearly, when they care full time for their partner with Alzheimer's disease, partners may experience significant feelings of loss much earlier than many people recognise (Loos and Bowd, 1997).

Feelings of loss and separation are experienced most severely by a partner when he or she can no longer connect with their partner in a real way — when, for example, a wife fails to recognise the presence of her own husband and children. This often, and understandably, causes much pain and grief, and intense and long-term comprehensive support services are needed during the specific stages of care (Gwyther *et al*, 1983; Grant *et al*, 1995).

The person with Alzheimer's disease tries to make sense of a world that is, for them, fragmented and forever disintegrating. In a very real sense their mental life is disappearing. Relatives often cling even to minor utterances, desperately trying to hang on to every lucid moment. In a very real sense the person people knew disappears and the experience of loss often creates fear and confusion for relatives. Children can become very upset when their parent or grandparent changes so radically. However, we know that emotional support, education and information can help (Morrissey, 1997).

Helping a person to express loss is only possible if the person is ready to do so and feels comfortable. Feelings of loss can often be explored during regular visits by a nurse as part of the care. Carers have multiple losses to contend with, and nurses must plan interventions to facilitate the process of pre-death grief for them. However, some caregivers may never completely resolve the pre-death and post-death losses that have resulted in caring for their relative (Liken and Collins, 1993).

Loss

I reached out my hand to my grandmother and tried to hold back the tears as I didn't know if I would ever see her again. Although she didn't understand the words, she did understand the feelings and we both cried.

(Relative)

There was a stage where we were all crying and Graham refused to leave his grandfather's bed even though his father and I wanted to shield him from the pain.

(Relative)

Alzheimer's disease can affect an individual's personal and social relationships profoundly. For those without experience as a carer, their initial understanding of Alzheimer's is often limited, given that many people with the disease can seem plausible in the early stages. Later, when the person is unable to function at home even with assistance, and is admitted to a nursing home for full-time or even respite care, some carers feel a sense of guilt, loss, relief and sometimes depression, as well as a feeling of abandonment. Many carers will go to extreme lengths to maintain communication, even though the person is devastated in the wake of dementia.

Some people, however, cannot bear the fact that their relatives have lost or are losing their cognitive abilities. Families all over the world have a story to tell about loss and the heartache of Alzheimer's disease in relation to the individual, their partner and family. It is also important to know that some sufferers are completely alone.

There is no shortage of theories explaining loss (Klein 1940; Lindemann, 1944; Kubler-Ross, 1970; Parkes, 1972). However many psychological and psychoanalytical theories, while offering useful insights, may seem quite detached and out of date in the everyday experiences of carers.

We need to be cautious about theories which talk about loss and provide a set of instructions on how to deal with it. Loss is complex, as are motives for caring, some of which make us question ourselves in many ways beyond the scope of media representations.

Psychological theories in relation to counselling and loss abound. Many contemporary theories tend to simplify loss into a neat set of stages or, most recently, into elaborate cognitive processes. The result is an ever-increasing array of competing theories, models and charts to guide the person through each step of counselling.

Anyone who has worked long hours as a carer and experienced the loss of a partner will understand that dealing with loss is different to theorising about it. Healing is not just about counselling a client, it is about caring and being with them through their ups and downs, including support for family, friends and relatives.

Nurses are undervalued in a similar way to carers by a society which often views their work as low priority. More importantly, a significant amount of care is in fact delivered by inexperienced and unqualified staff. Recent community care initiatives may mean that more older people are at risk from abuse by their carers (Wilson, 1993). Sadly, much of the care work in nursing homes and hospitals places great emphasis on physical care, the result being that psychological care and emotional support frequently remain virtually unaddressed. This means that many carers have to deal with care-giving and loss on their own. If care regresses to containment, the freedom and quality of care of the whole person is significantly reduced. Nurses are not set apart in the same way that doctors are which means that the medical model continues to have significant power in practice (James and Field, 1996).

More funding and resources need to be invested in elderly care and directed especially to the carers and nurses who are dealing directly with the effects of Alzheimer's disease on the person and their family. Many of the factors that can help people living with the reality of Alzheimer's disease are beyond the grasp of a traditional medical model, particularly in relation to caring: being with a person; quality of life; spiritual, psychological and emotional support; listening and responding to the everyday experiences of carers in full-time care.

Medicine very often has an inadequate understanding of effective communication with clients (Fallowfield, 1992) and the qualities that are required in being with a client. Alzheimer's disease brings multiple losses and the early ones are perhaps the most profound and difficult because affected individuals still have enough cognitive function to understand and feel horrified by what is happening to them; to face the painful realisation of losing their minds and those they love dearly as they drift into Alzheimer's disease. Early losses are also very hard and painful for caregivers as they are still trying to come to terms with the meaning of the diagnosis and the desperate reality of a future dominated by the demands of care-giving. Many carers also have other caring demands, including children and a partner (Hicks, 1988), and competing care demands can cause conflict in the family.

Some of the specific losses facing a person with Alzheimer's are: retiring from work; handing over personal affairs; loss of cognitive functioning; loss of contact with reality; sometimes loss of love and affection; loss of control of basic physical activities such as housework, food preparation, shopping, using the telephone, finance; loss of control of body functions such as toileting; and loss of identity of self and others.

A most profound loss is surely loss of independence. It is a difficult and painful reality when a person has to leave both home and familiar surroundings and move in with a loved one or be admitted to a nursing home.

Theory

Various counselling approaches have been put forward to help people to deal with loss and grief (Carl Rogers, 1984; Worden, 1982; Raphael, 1984; Parkes, 1981), while other texts address the counselling of older people (Scrutton, 1995). However, many theories fail to integrate the effect of being with a person and their family on a day-to-day basis, as opposed to a few consultations.

Carers, too, may lack close emotional bonds with friends and family, and social support may decline the more deeply they become immersed in caring. Such a lack of support is not uncommon in the community (Bodnar *et al*, 1994).

> *In many cases it takes a life crisis, such as a loss or a move for us to recognise our need for our own love, concern and support. As important as it is to take care of ourselves every day, our need for self-support and self-concern is critical when we are grieving. If we neglect ourselves at such times we impede our recovery.*

(Tatelbaum, 1981)

In part this may be true, but the factors influencing self-neglect are to some extent due to the burden of care and social isolation. Many carers caring for a relative at home recognise they sometimes neglect their own needs for those of others. It is impossible in a few lines to convey the demands of day-to-day care. However, such experiences are important for understanding how we can improve the crisis of caring.

Much of the work of nurses in elderly care aims to deliver effective physical and social care, and helps to promote positive coping strategies for client and carers. It has been suggested that counselling can help people to recognise the importance of self-love and self-care (Scrutton, 1995).

In the early stages of Alzheimer's disease it is important to help carers and relatives to understand the entire picture, including the progression, of Alzheimer's disease. This task is sometimes avoided or neglected by professionals, but it is important to educate, to identify gaps in understanding and to give information so that carers and families can be assisted in making realistic decisions about care. It is important to work with carers to enable their understanding of issues surrounding assessment, diagnosis, treatment and care, social support, counselling, finance and legal issues.

Multiple losses are part of the course of Alzheimer's disease and loss of function is a dramatic part of the illness for the person. Understanding loss through loss of function is often a useful first step.

Understanding the effect of brain degeneration and loss of function

Although the cells in the human body are clearly dying from birth, premature brain death is undesirable and generally considered by medicine to be unusual. Dementia of the Alzheimer's type robs people of their normal brain life; the degeneration is progressive and the prognosis poor.

For many people the ultimate loss is the loss of their brain function. Perhaps this is so because the brain is what controls our every thought and movement. Loss of control is most undesirable, but even more disturbing is the degeneration of basic brain functions such as memory, perception and other cognitive functions.

Brain degeneration or loss of function is disturbing in a number of ways which are beyond the focus of medicine. Alzheimer's disease has no cure and therefore the medical model is, to a large extent, redundant — more so, perhaps, because this disease affects mainly older people. The elderly have never held centre stage for medicine or society and are also negatively portrayed by an ageist culture.

There is some public recognition that there is no treatment, no miracle drug, no technological or research breakthrough visible (Feely, 1997), and this casts despair and lack of hope. Such a disease crushes the myth of the miracle of medicine and/or science. There is a very real loss to society of the disappearing lives of people, many of whom were especially gifted but all of whom are special to their families.

Many of the people who have Alzheimer's disease have lived independent lives. As a result, many experience loss of independence, and a growing dependence on others. Furthermore, the personal life of their partner is invaded, given that they are often their primary carer too.

Recently John Bayley, literary critic and former Warton professor of English at Oxford University, has discussed caring for his wife, Iris Murdoch, a famous Irish writer who recently died from Alzheimer's disease (Bayley cited in Petty, 1998). It is clear that he, too, found it difficult to express publicly the dreadful feelings of loss and despair he felt. More than this, he conveyed a truly admirable respect, patience and love of caring for his wife.

The fog of Alzheimer's disease began closing in around Dame Iris, now seventy-nine, several years ago: by 1996 there was no doubt about the diagnosis. The gradual atrophy that produced twenty-six novels of great erudition, has left Bayley scrabbling around to adjust to the narrowed perimeters of their lives, with Dame Iris trailing blankly, if benignly in his wake.

Her co-ordination is failing, and worse, she cannot grasp the concept of the simplest of activities, like dressing or washing the dishes. 'She can do her shoelaces, but doesn't get around to it. The fact is the one big thing has gone', murmurs Bayley aged seventy-three. 'Nothing else mattered but her writing'. Her last novel, Jackson's Dilemma, *was published in 1995.*

'By the time the reviews came out, she was unable to understand them. I puzzle over it every day I don't think she realises what she has lost.' As a result of loss of function John Bayley decribes his present state as a 'gentlemanly confinement'. 'I have to make sure the doors are locked all the time. Several times she has wandered off quite a distance, crossing roads and so on. Once she was missing for five hours and I had to call the police. It's impossible to be separated. She gets upset if I leave her with anyone.'

'When she falls into a depression I have to take her for a walk around the block. When we go shopping she is happy to

sit in the car and watch the people go past. It is very difficult to go to restaurants. The last time we went some months ago, it was embarrassing to put it mildly. Instead of popping out to the loo, she decided to do it on the spot. A perfectly natural thing when you think of animals, but traumatic for the waiters.'

Other times when I prepare to leave, Iris tries to hand me her jacket. 'That's your jacket darling,' says Bayley lightly. I thank her for her inscription on my book. She looks at the volume as if it were a foreign object, then puts her arms around me and utters a tinkling cry: 'A-a-a-ah'.

(Bayley cited in: Petty, 1998)

The horrors of caring for people with Alzheimer's disease present many more disturbing accounts of caring — an ongoing story which may remain hidden and unnoticed in institutional care, including nursing homes. However, such loss must be recognised by society and not banished or hidden from the public.

The quality of care for people with or affected by Alzheimer's disease is surely a marker of a civilised society. I have experienced caring both personally and professionally. Reflecting on such experiences is important.

One day I arrived on an elderly care ward in a local hospital. I noticed two women trying to get out of the ward. The staff brought them back. This happened again and again and both the staff and these women were very distressed. I was told the women had Alzheimer's disease. The lasting impact of that visit for me was the fact that I was free to leave but the staff and patients were confined. This situation reminded me of purgatory; a perpetual place of suffering. I felt a great sense of sadness for all concerned. It is important to question such experiences in order to find ways to comfort people in such extremely distressing situations.

When you are afraid, who comforts you? If there is no one there, what will you do? Ask? But if you have Alzheimer's disease you may be unable to ask. Your needs must be met by a carer. It is at this profound stage that we must dig deep into our consciousness and recognise how much we depend on the kindness and care of others. It is easy to blame the inability of others, but surely we must foster hope and caring, and show how each one of us can make a difference. We depend totally on the compassion and kindness of others in the late stages of Alzheimer's disease.

For those who care on a regular basis for a person with Alzheimer's disease, it is evident that this area is profoundly difficult. It is not always respected and can be a very lonely experience for nurses and carers. Care and loss is central to all human and animal life. Birth itself is sometimes experienced as a loss to a woman, and caring as an inevitable part of being a mother.

However, though the majority of carers in the UK continue to be women, caring is not and should not be seen as being exclusive to women (Pitkeathley, 1995). No matter how much care we provide for a human or an animal, loss is inevitable as is death. So it is with Alzheimer's disease. Carers involved in caring for people with the disease may not always recognise that loss is a central theme in their daily lives. Sometimes, as a result of being so familiar, they may not always be acutely aware of changes in the person with Alzheimer's.

In examining issues around loss, the needs of children are often forgotten as is the valuable contribution children can make to the quality of life of a person with Alzheimer's disease.

Education and support for children

It is exteremely difficult to prepare a relative or partner for the magnitude of human suffering, disintegration and loss involved in caring for an individual with Alzheimer's disease. It is also especially important to offer education and support for children, who have special needs in adjusting to profound and often distressing changes in a relative. In addition, staff in hospitals and nursing homes must recognise the fear that such environments can create in a child or adolescent.

When a child visits a nursing home, the time should be planned and managed in a way that demonstrates sensitivity to the individual child and should include some education given by the staff in a simple and friendly manner. Children can benefit from reading about Alzheimer's disease and, where possible, should be encouraged to do so. Older children can also watch simple and non-threatening educational videos. To a large extent, the success of such strategies depends on forming a close, trusting relationship with the child. Care delivered with compassion, love and sensitivity continues to be the basic language in dementia care, however we dress it up.

Children, like adults, may need supportive counselling or special support during a family bereavement. Working with several family members together can be useful both in helping children to access any emotional support available and in making family members more sensitive to individual children. Painting and music can assist children in the expression of feelings. Regular meetings with the family can enable professionals, such as nurses, to be more readily accepted, especially when visiting at home.

Education programmes in Canada show how effective education can be. When Cathi Gorham-Mol found her son crying on the couch after visiting his grandfather, she asked what was wrong. 'Grandpa doesn't love me any more; he didn't hug me goodbye,' she recalls Lucas, then five, saying. 'He didn't mean to forget,' Mrs Gorham-Mol explained to her son who was close to his grandfather and noticed with pain the changes Alzheimer's disease had wrought. That incident, more than a year ago, was a turning point not only for that Woodstock, Ontario mother, but also for several parents of school-aged children grappling with a grandparent's dementia.

The result has been 'Remember Me', a programme offered by the Alzheimer's Society of Oxford in Southwest Ontario. It brings children, aged seven to fourteen, together to learn about what Alzheimer's does to the brain, how memory and behaviour are affected and how they, as grandchildren, can cope with the changes they see but can't always explain (Lipovenko, 1998). Working in this area is in part accepting that love and loss are shared experiences by many families, partners and friends.

For experienced carers, who are often family members or partners, it is clear that emotional support and understanding are required during and after the process of care. However, individual professional support is frequently in short supply (Scrutton, 1995) and is substituted by carers' groups (Yale, 1995). In many nursing homes, carers groups are one form of support system where staff and relatives can express their ongoing concerns.

I don't know what I would have done without this carers' group at Darland House. The people have been so kind to me and my wife. They know what I was going through and they listen.

(Carer)

To love a person and watch them disintegrate in body, mind and spirit has many consequences outside the parameters of this discussion. However, some extracts from carers are useful:

Well, I have been married for over forty years. We did

everything together, the shopping and everything. The house feels empty. I feel guilty for leaving her here and it seems so long until I see her again. She doesn't know me but still I like to be there. I am sad as I know what she was like before and yes I miss her.

(Carer)

There were the special things she did that made her my mother. Each day caring for her I would remember going for walks together, laughing, sharing silly things, being together. Sometimes in the past I would confide in her and she responded as my special friend. She understood me like no other could and her life and our special friendship was disappearing as a medical diagnosis of Alzheimer's disease was being made.

(Carer)

When the diagnosis came I was uncertain in disbelief. I cared for her with the help of my family. I cried so many times, mostly in private; the pain, the burden, was so unbearable so all-embracing. Sometimes I couldn't sleep. Eventually day by day the mother I knew and loved died. I continued to care for her. I felt guilty that I was not caring for my husband and family. I can't explain my feelings the loss was unbearable, I grieved but felt guilty knowing that she was still alive and needing care. I felt guilty for having my own feelings when she had Alzheimer's disease, my mother who was so gentle, it isn't fair.

(Carer)

There may also be a blurring of personal boundaries between the caregiver and client which can result in a loss of personal space or self-esteem, and sometimes in family conflict. For the carer there may also be a loss of time available to spend with other family members and friends. For partners there is often a need to be with their partner, and a need or desire to care for them. For a professional carer, the motivation to care may be in relation to duty or a task (Campbell, 1984). However, regardless of status, a person cannot share in such a real human experience of loss, unless they themselves have loved and experienced loss on some level.

In caring for a person with Alzheimer's disease, a carer needs practical support: day services, social support, GP contact, a carers' group, transport, and good social networks to name but a few. Frequently the caregiver feels overwhelmed and taken over by the needs of the person in care (Loos and Bowd, 1997), and depression is not uncommon (Collins *et al*, 1994).

Bereavement and loss are multidimensional, and in Alzheimer's disease the process is twofold; occurring firstly during care-giving and secondly after death (Jones and Martinson, 1992). Alzheimer's disease has been described as a 'living bereavement' (Taylor, 1987), however for many carers this kind of physical, psychological, emotional and spiritual loss also puts them in touch with other past and current losses. The process, therefore, is perhaps more accurately described as a 'raw wound' rather than a 'living bereavement'. Some caregivers may never completely resolve the pre-death and post-death losses that have resulted in caring for their relative (Liken and Collins, 1993). There is a real need to develop grief and bereavement services in specific relation to Alzheimer's disease (Murphy et al, 1997).

Both religion and culture have important influences on when and how grief is expressed. However, having the love and compassion of a friend or social support system should not be assumed at such times. Alzheimer's disease creates multiple losses including loss of function in relation to a person's psychology, physical and social abilities. There are also changes in sensory functions, eventually leading to increased dependence.

The task of caring falls primarily upon a few relatives and friends, often, in turn, decreasing their own social support networks (Hicks, 1988; Warner, 1995). Professional assistance is sometimes sparse, or even non-existent, and as a result, carers face the problem of coping on their own when dealing with the trauma which the course of Alzheimer's creates (Scrutton, 1995).

Three years later, I am better able to understand the damage that was done to John, to me, to our family and friends through ignorance about dementia — my own ignorance, and also that of John's GP. That ignorance perpetuated my own confusion, guilt and inability to believe that I was capable of doing anything positive. John's disintegration was a threat to my own integrity: accepting that this was so has brought the opportunity to understand a great deal about myself, and in so doing to improve my relationships with those around me. Watching the disintegration of somebody close and experiencing it within yourself is painful, but in the end all the anguish need not be a waste.

(Forsythe, 1993)

Avenues of support

There are many avenues of support through professional agencies and day centres, and through voluntary agencies such as Age Concern, the Alzheimer's Disease Society, and others whose addresses are given at the back of this book. Counselling may be one avenue of support, however more and more services are setting up support groups for carers. Some of the areas that can be dealt with in such groups include the many issues surrounding diagnosis and treatment, and dealing with the changed person, including difficult behaviour.

Many homes now offer respite care for both the person with Alzheimer's disease and their carer. Some care homes also offer a counselling service on a specific day where carers can discuss their own adjustment to care-giving. More importantly, counselling can help the person to prepare for bereavement and adjust to changes that result from Alzheimer's disease, including working through thoughts and feelings, family support and health promotion (Young, 1996). It is also important to facilitate access to hospice care, which should be encouraged particularly for families caring for a relative in the end stages of Alzheimer's disease and residing in nursing home facilities (Murphy *et al*, 1997). As has been discussed, education is also vital for carers and there are now programmes in universities and colleges specifically aimed at carers in relation to dementia care. Information can also be found on the Internet.

As professionals we may not always recognise the need to work closely with people who are dealing with caring, change and multiple loss. It is my hope that recognition for the work of carers and respect for the needs of the elderly, including those with dementia, will increase. Carers have basic rights to support during and after care-giving and, furthermore, education and support must reach children who often have their own specific needs in these circumstances. I leave you with a quote from a carer which expresses the totality of the loss of a partner with Alzheimer's disease:

*There is just you and the silence and the absence of all you
have lived for, all you have loved, all that is special, there is
no comfort really.*

(Partner)

References

Aronson E (1988) *The Social Animal*, 5th edn. Freeman & Company, New
York

Bayley J In: Petty M (1998) Alzheimer's Disease. *The Times Weekend* 12
Sept

Bodnar JC, Kiecolt G, Janice K (1994) Caregiver depression after
bereavement: Chronic stress isn't over when it's over. *Psychol Aging*
9(3): 372–80

Bowlby J (1980) *Attachment and loss.Vol. 3: Loss, sadness and depression.*
Basic Books, New York

Campbell AV (1984) *Moderated love: A Theology of Professional Care.*
Holy Trinity Church, Marylebone Road, London

Collins C, Stommel M, Wang, S et al (1994) Caregiving transitions:
changes in depression among family caregivers of relatives with
dementia. *Nurs Res* **43**(4): 220–5

Dyson J (1997) The meaning of spirituality: a literature review. *J Adv Nurs*
26(6): 1183–8

Fallowfield L (1992) The ideal consultation. *Br J Hosp Med* **47**:
364–7

Feely J (1997) Alzheimer's Disease. *Health Which?*:172–3

Forsythe E (1990) *Alzheimer's Disease: the long bereavement.* Faber &
Faber, London

Grant L (1998) *Remind me who I am again.* Granta, London

Grant LA, Kane RA, Stark AJ (1995) Beyond labels: nursing home care for
Alzheimer's disease in and out of special care units. *J Am Ger Soc*
43(5): 569–76

Gwyther LP, Matteson MA (1983) Care for the caregivers. *J Gerontological
Nurs* **9**(2): 92–5

Heyman B (1995) *Researching user perspectives on community healthcare.*
Chapman & Hall, London

Hicks C (1988) *Who cares?* Virago Press Ltd, London

Iverson L (1988) The Neurobiology of Ageing. The fifty-seventh Stephen
Memorial Lecture. *Conquest* (178): 1-12

James V, Field D (1996) Who holds the power? Some problems and issues
affecting the nursing care of dying patients. *Eur J Cancer Nurs* **5**:
73–80

Jones PS, Martinson IM (1992) The experience of bereavement in
caregivers of family members with Alzheimer's disease. *Image J Nurs
Sch* **24**(3): 172–6

Klein M (1940) Mourning and its relationship to manic-depressive states.
Int J Psychoanal **21**:125–53

Kreiner A (1995) After hours. Nurse hopes book will help others whose loved ones have disappeared. *Nurseweek* **8**(14):22: 10–23

Kubler-Ross E (1970) *On death and dying.* Tavistock, London

Liken MA, Collins CE (1993) Grieving: facilitating the process for dementia caregivers. *Psychosocial Nursing & Mental Health Services.* **31**(1): 21–6; 30–1

Lindemann C (1944) The symptomatology and management of acute grief. *Am J Psychiatry* **124**:1190–5

Lipovenko D (1998) Alzhcimer's course helps grandchildren. *The Globe and Mail* Woodstock, Ontario: 1

Loos C, Bowd A (1997) Caregivers of persons with Alzheimer's disease: some neglected implications of the experience of personal loss and grief. *Death studies* **21**(5): 501–14

Mace N, Rabins P (1991) *The 36-Hour Day.* The John Hopkins University Press, Baltimore, Maryland, USA

Morrissey M (1997) A survey of information provision in mental health: What have we learned? *Int J Psychiatric Nurs Res* **3** (3): 361–9

Morrissey M, Hill RG (1997) The costs of formal and informal caring in mental health. *Ment Health Nurs* **17**(5): 12–3

Murphy K, Hanrahan P, Luchins D (1997) A survey of grief and bereavement in nursing homes: the importance of hospice grief and bereavement for the end-stage of Alzheimer's disease patient and family. *J Am Ger Soc* **45**(9): 1104–7

Ogg J, Bennett G (1992) Elder Abuse in Britain.*Br Med J* **305**(24): 998–9

Parkes CM (1972) *Bereavement: studies of grief in adult life.* International Universities Press, New York

Parkes CM (1981) Evaluation of bereavement service. *J Preventive Psychiatry* **1**:179–88

Pickles H (1998) Caring for the elderly: part two. You're not born to sacrifice your life to look after your parents. *You Magazine, Mail on Sunday,* Associated Newspapers Ltd, London, June: 42–7

Pitkeathley J (1995) *It's my duty isn't it? The plight of carers in our society.* Souvenir Press Limited. London

Raphael B (1984) *The anatomy of bereavement: a handbook for the caring professions.* Hutchinson, London

Rogers C (1984) *Client-centred therapy.* Constable, London

Scrutton S (1995) *Bereavement and Grief: supporting older people through loss.* Edward Arnold, London

Tatelbaum J (1981) *The courage to grieve: creating living, recovery and growth through grief.* Heinemann, London

Taylor B (1987) The confused elderly: a living bereavement Alzheimer's disease. *Nurs Times* **83**(30): 27–30

Warner N (1995) *Better tomorrows.* National Association of Carers, London

Wilson G (1993) Disclosing the truth about grannie bashing. In: Family Policy Studies Centre Bulletin, June: 4–5

Worden JW (1982) *Grief counselling and grief therapy.* Tavistock, London and New York

Yale R (1995) *Developing Support Groups for Individuals With Early-Stage Alzheimer's Disease.* Health Professions Press Inc., PO Box 10624, Baltimore, MD 21285-0624

Young K (1996) Health, health promotion and the elderly. *J Clin Nurs* **5**(4): 241–8

5

Legal and financial issues

James Robinson and Matthew V Morrissey

In Alzheimer's disease difficult transitions have to be made and control of financial and legal affairs may of necessity have to be transferred to another person.

(Robinson and Morrissey, 1999)

Introduction

Due to the nature of the illness, many Alzheimer's sufferers become increasingly less able to manage their own legal and financial affairs or to make appropriate decisions about their care. When such situations occur, people with Alzheimer's need others to make decisions for them, and to take responsibility for the financial and legal implications of their disease.

Treatment and control

The law usually upholds the right of a person to decide what shall be done with his or her own body, and any action which involves the threat or use of force (however slight) upon a person is deemed unlawful unless there is consent or some legal justification for acting without it.

Apart from an emergency, when it may not be possible to obtain a person's consent, a patient's agreement is normally required before he or she may be admitted to hospital and given treatment.

The main exceptions to this rule are compulsory admissions to hospital or other types of residential care under Section 47 of the National Assistance Act, 1948, and compulsory admissions to hospital under Sections 2 and 3 of the Mental Health Act, 1983.

Compulsory admission to residential care

Section 47 of the National Assistance Act, 1948, permits a person to be compulsorily removed from where they are living and taken to a place where they will receive 'the necessary care and attention'. The grounds for proceeding under the Act have three components:

1   That the person is suffering from grave chronic disease or, being aged, infirm or physically incapacitated, is living in unsanitary conditions.

2   That the person is unable to devote care to him or herself and is not receiving from other persons proper care and attention.

3   That his or her removal from home is necessary, either in his or her own interest or for preventing injury to the health of, or serious nuisance to others.

The wording of Section 47 is narrowly prescriptive. The procedure is initiated by the community physician who certifies in writing to the district local authority that the grounds exist. (Note that in the non-unitary authorities, the district local authority is not the local social services authority which is responsible for providing residential care and services to people in their own homes.) The local authority may then apply to the magistrates' court for an order to remove the person to a suitable hospital or other place.

It is important to note that an order under Section 47 relates solely to the person's removal and detention elsewhere. It does not give authority for a person to be treated without his or her consent.

Applications under Section 47 must be made after giving the person concerned seven days' notice, 'or to some person in charge of him' or her (note that this does not necessarily mean the nearest relative or next of kin) seven days' notice. However, an emergency procedure is made available by the National Assistance (Amendment) Act 1951, in cases where the person fulfils conditions 1 and 2 above, and where it is necessary to move the person in his or her own interests and without delay. In such cases it is not obligatory to give notice.

Compulsory admission to hospital

Relatively few applications are made under the National Assistance Act compared with the number of compulsory admissions to hospital under the Mental Health Act, 1983. The process whereby a person may be 'sectioned' (an unfortunate word which carries with it connotations of compulsion and stigma), that is admitted to hospital compulsorily for assessment or treatment, does not involve any application to a court. Most compulsory admissions are made by the patient's nearest relative or an approved social worker (ASW) and supported by one or two doctors. If accepted by the hospital to which it is addressed, the application itself is authority to detain and usually to treat the patient without his or her consent.

Under Section 2, an application for admission for assessment authorises the patient's detention for up to 28 days. The application must be supported by the recommendations of two doctors (one of whom is approved under the Act) to the effect that the patient is suffering from mental disorder of a nature and degree which warrants his or her detention in a hospital for assessment and that he or she needs to be so detained in the interests of his or her own health or safety, or with a view to the protection of other persons.

Under Section 3, an application for admission for treatment may again be made either by the nearest relative or an approved social worker. Importantly, if the patient's nearest relative objects to the admission, the social worker must apply to the court to displace the relative in order to proceed. The patient may be detained in the first instance for up to six months, and there is a procedure through which the detention may be renewed.

Consent

The Mental Health Act provides for informal admissions to hospital, that is, at the patient's request or with his or her consent. The wording of the Act merits consideration (author's insertion within brackets). Section 131 provides:

> *Nothing* [in the 1983 Act] *shall be construed as preventing a patient who required treatment for mental disorder from being admitted to any hospital without any application, or direction rendering him liable to being detained under* [the] *Act.*

This was in identical terms to Section 5 of the 1959 Mental Health Act which had been enacted to implement the recommendations of the

Royal Commission on the Law relating to Mental Illness and Mental Deficiency (1957), that the law (author's emphasis in bold):

> *should be altered, in relation to all forms of mental disorder, by abandoning the assumption that compulsory powers must be used unless the patient can express a positive desire for treatment and replacing this by the offer of care, without deprivation of liberty, to all who need it and are* **not unwilling** *to receive it.*

> (Mental Health Act, 1959)

All hospitals providing psychiatric treatment should be free to admit patients for any length of time without any legal formality and without power to detain.

The state of the present law concerning 'consent' and 'informal admissions' was carefully considered by the House of Lords in what has become known as the 'Bournewood case'. In what has become the definitive interpretation of the law, Regina v Bournewood Community and Mental Health NHS Trust Ex parte L (1998), it was determined that the basis upon which a hospital is entitled to treat and care for persons who are admitted as informal patients but lack the capacity to consent to such treatment or care, is the common law doctrine of necessity, which has the effect of justifying actions which might otherwise be unlawful.

The role of the nearest relative

The role of the 'nearest relative' is acknowledged in the Mental Health Act which obliges the approved social worker to inform the nearest relative of an admission and of his or her right to discharge the patient. This must be done 'within a reasonable time'.

However, if an ASW is proposing to make an application for a patient's long-term admission for treatment, he or she must consult the person who appears to be the nearest relative. The only exceptions are where this is not reasonably practicable, or where this would involve unreasonable delay. Whether or not the nearest relative has been consulted, he or she has the right subsequently to prevent an admission for treatment. In such a situation, the county court has the power to displace the nearest relative if it is satisfied that the nearest relative objects unreasonably to the application for admission for treatment.

Definition of 'nearest relative'

The Mental Health Act defines 'nearest relative' by taking whoever comes first on the list of relatives in the following order:

- husband or wife
- son or daughter
- father or mother
- brother or sister
- grandparent
- grandchild
- uncle or aunt
- nephew or niece.

If there is more than one in the same category, the elder is preferred regardless of gender. However, any relative who is caring for the patient or with whom the relative usually resides is promoted to the top of the list.

People whose parents were not married to one another are regarded as related only to their mother's side of the family and not to their father unless he has 'parental responsibility'. A father obtains parental responsibility either by obtaining a court order to that effect or by a parental responsibility agreement with the mother.

Anyone who lives outside the UK is automatically ignored, as is a person under 18 years of age unless that person is the patient's husband or wife. The list ends with any person who is not a relative within any of the above categories, but with whom the patient ordinarily resides and has done so continuously for five years.

Enduring powers of attorney

An ordinary power of attorney is a document by which one person (the donor) authorises another (the donee) to act on his or her behalf. To be effective it must be signed by the donor and witnessed.

In circumstances where people would like to appoint their own agent in case they should become incapable of managing their own affairs when their faculties fail, an ordinary power of attorney is not appropriate because a power of attorney is automatically revoked when the donor becomes incapable of being contacted.

In 1983, the Law Commission proposed a scheme which was eventually enacted in the Enduring Powers of Attorney Act, 1985. Under this Act an enduring power of attorney can be created which has the advantage of not being affected by the subsequent incapability in the donor.

An enduring power of attorney can be created validly only by a donor with sufficient mental capacity to do so. There are three basic safeguards which safeguard the donor:

1   The power must be granted on a prescribed form which incorporates an explanation of its effect.

2   Once the attorney (donee) has reason to believe that the donor is or is becoming mentally incapable of managing his or her property and affairs, the donee must apply to register the enduring power of attorney (EPA) with the Court of Protection. The donee must notify both the donor and his or her relatives of this application.

3   The wording of the power of attorney form should be carefully noted and pains should be taken to explain to the donor the consequences of signing the document. The effect of registration is that the Court of Protection has power to give directions on the management of property and the affairs of the donor.

The duties of the attorney are confined to the conduct of financial and business affairs. An EPA is not capable of providing authority in the matter of the donor's welfare; it cannot be used to authorise or forbid medical treatments or personal care decisions .

The advantages of an EPA are many; the donor can choose the attorney he or she trusts, to act as he or she would have wished and can give the chosen person general or precise instructions as he or she thinks fit. Once obtained, a copy of the power of attorney will normally be sent to the donor's bank, enabling the attorney to manage the bank accounts and other assets in accordance with the donor's wishes. This will enable settlement of debts and liabilities as they become due.

The Court of Protection

Another procedure for protecting the interests of an Alzheimer sufferer ('mentally incapable person') is to involve the powers of the Court of

Protection which has considerable powers to act in relation to the property and affairs of the patient.

Any person can apply to the Court of Protection to have a patient's property placed under the Court's jurisdiction on the grounds that the patient is incapable of managing his or her own affairs. A relative, a director of social services, a creditor, adviser or friend may make the application. The application form (supplied by the Court) must be accompanied by a medical certificate which states that the person is incapable, by reason of mental disorder, of managing his or her own affairs.

The Court's powers are extensive and include selling, dealing with or disposing of the patient's property, making settlements or gifts on the patient's behalf, making a will, dissolving a patient's partnership, reimbursing any person who has previously paid the patient's debts, and conducting legal proceedings on the patient's behalf.

Conclusion

This provides a summary of the legal position of a person suffering from a mental disorder (the expression 'mental disorder' includes 'mental illness' and, by definition, Alzheimer's disease) with regard to his or her treatment (voluntary or compulsory) and care. If the sufferer is willing to delegate responsibility under a power of attorney, the financial management of his or her affairs can best be dealt with when the disease is in its early stages. The donee, who is usually a family member, will then be able to deal with all financial matters including, as is often the case, selling the donor's property in order to pay for his or her continuing care.

In those cases where a power of attorney is inappropriate, for example where the sufferer is not competent to understand the nature and purpose of the document, the remedy is to apply to the Court of Protection which will take responsibility for the patient's affairs.

The financial and legal status of the sufferer is not usually the most immediately pressing of the carer's concerns. However, a background knowledge of the law can provide some reassurance for the carer when coping with a disease in a loved one which can, at times, be both distressing and emotionally taxing. Surprisingly, the law can sometimes be a friend.

Further reading

Cretney SM (1991) *Enduring Powers of Attorney: A Practitioner's Guide.* 3rd edn, Jordan, Bristol

Griffiths A, Roberts G (1995) *The Law and Elderly People.* 2nd edn, Routledge, London

Hogget B (1996) *Mental Health Law.* 4th edn, Sweet and Maxwell, London

Jones R (1983) *Mental Health Act Manual.* 5th edn, Sweet and Maxwell: London

Social Services Inspectorate (1990) *Caring for Quality: Guidelines on Standards for Residential Homes for Elderly People.* HMSO, London

6

The experience of care

Mary Morrissey, Jane Webborn, Elizabeth Robinson and Anonymous

The change started at the age of sixty-eight years, just after my dad died, so I thought it was due to his loss, but if I only knew something about Alzheimer's disease I could have made life much better for my mum.

(Mary Morrissey)

It seemed to confirm some unspoken fears that all was not well. A curtain seemed to be coming across which had been clear from the look of confusion which covered their father's face. This could be what is called the invisible side of Alzheimer's.

(Jane Webborn)

Visiting her in the mental health unit was so traumatic because we always dreaded leaving her, she wanted to come with us... the guilt and sadness in these moments was dreadful.

(Elizabeth Robinson)

It was so easy also for me to assume when looking at her blank, increasingly expressionless face, that she did not care about what was happening to her.

(Anonymous)

'If only I knew': *Mary Morrissey*

My best friend, who happens to be my mother, a smart, caring, gentle, loving mother and person, great cook, home maker, listener, never judgmental, always cheerful and fun loving. Mother of eleven children who worked very hard and spent some time in hospital with ill health.

The change started at the age of sixty-eight years, just after my dad died, so I thought it was due to his loss, but if I only knew something about Alzheimer's disease I could have made life much better for my mum.

I suppose looking back it started happening very slowly. One of the first things which started me wondering was my mother and myself were very close and I knew she was always great to keep secrets, so I always confided in her. It was a big secret I told her and I found out she had told someone, who I knew she would never dream of telling, as this person could not keep a secret and my mother knew this, so I was very upset but I knew then that my mother was changing. At this time she got ill with flu and I stayed with her, it was a hard Christmas. When she would normally have her Christmas baking done I found some tins with Christmas cakes wrapped in tin foil. She said she had her baking finished — six cakes. I opened one up, and of course they were soda cakes — all gone mildew. I was really upset, other signs were that she was not using the washing machine, but hand washing. This would be how she would have washed when we were young.

Also when it was bedtime, her nature, which was always the same, had changed. She was always reading leaflets which were on a table for years with her rosary beads. The leaflets were gone and she had broken her rosary beads. As she was a very tidy person I found it strange that she was putting her clothes under her mattress. Nothing was the same any more about my mum. I noticed a strange look on her face and she didn't smile like she always did and had very little conversation. I thought I would take her to the doctor as I thought she didn't look well. The doctor told me my mother was depressed, I was very shocked, as my mother was always very cheerful; it was something so new.

I noticed other signs when I visited her she would tell me about things that she thought were happening. I realised my mother was telling me about people in a programme on television she was watching, that she thought was real. On a later visit I realised she was losing weight, when I asked what she was eating she could list off a lot of meals she had, but her fridge told another story — weeks of shopping left untouched. My sister started giving her her dinner as I lived a long way from her and I was working full time. When I saw her during this time she complained about the dinners and said she didn't want to have them again. I thought my mum had changed so much.

I was feeling very disappointed and cross at her and would tell her so. She would deny saying those things and would say in her usual caring voice 'take no notice'.

Gradually the television she loved was not turned on and she looked vacant. I would scold her for not eating and ask her to come and stay with me, but my mother loved her home — if I only knew I would have stayed with her for a few nights a week. But I still, in spite of all the signs, thought my mother knew what she was doing. Oh how this hurts today.

One day things changed for ever. I visited my mum with my sister who had not seen her for quite some time was shocked with what she saw. Her sitting at the empty fireplace having obviously lost so much weight. We got her ready and brought her to live with us. She was very much loved by my children and husband and she was settled after some time of wandering around at night. She started imaginary sewing, but all the time she would be ripping at her skirt. I tried to stop her doing this as I felt her hands were so tired from all the activity. She got very cross at television programmes sometimes and gradually we all knew granny was quite normal at times and was really different other times.

She was in the early stages of Alzheimer's disease, this was a new word to me, I had heard of people being senile, but not this. So I got on with looking after mum, but of course doing all the wrong things, like when she would dry the washing up with me and kept putting the cups back into the water and would say someone else had done it. I would say 'but mother you are the one doing this'. Also, she would look out of the window and say that it is someone looking in at us, but I would say I did not see anyone. She would feed the dog with her dinner, put cushions on the hot range, but when my grandchild came in she would love to feed and play with her and she was her usual gentle self.

I think the saddest day for me was that my mother was a wonderful hand writer. Her handwriting was always admired by people. I asked her to write a letter to my brother in England and I couldn't believe what I saw — I cried that day. Some weeks after this she got very restless and agitated and wanted to go home. I took her home, but there was no response at all and, she barely responded to the grandchildren who lived next to her. It was at this time my mother was so insistent on going home that she would get very upset when I would say 'you can't go home'. Sadly she said she was really upset because her mother would be worried about her not being home. I would be trying to stop her telling her that her mother was dead. This was a continuous battle after some more crying she settled, but at this time she would need watching all the time. How difficult it was not to be able to talk to my mother, sometimes she would make sense, but those times got shorter.

My husband and myself decided we would take mother to the seaside for a holiday as she loved the seaside. We stayed in an hotel but my mother didn't notice she was at the seaside. I tried to get her to look at the beautiful sandy shore and the sea but she just looked vacant and shook her head. She played at her food in the hotel and people would keep looking and in the end I was glad to take my mother home.

I noticed at this time her family visits were getting less and less and in the end I was the total carer. My mother was still gentle and loved to be cuddled. At this time she also started wetting herself and didn't know when to use the toilet, also she was unable to wash herself and didn't know which part of clothing went where, but knew how to button her cardigan, tie up her shoes and she loved it when I would put her make up on and her watch on. She kept losing her rings and also her watch, so because she had lost her wedding ring I put it in a safe place. My mother had reached the stage that she was incontinent and needed help washing and feeding. I also found it a big ordeal to take her to the hairdresser, although I knew she liked it, but sometimes she was just so nervous about it all.

It took seven years for my mother to reach this stage. The winter of 1995 I took a decision not to have my mother injected for flu as she had the flu injection a few years previously and developed pneumonia, but my mother got the flu and it did develop into pneumonia. My mother, before she died, looked for her wedding ring and knew all the family by name and yet two of the years I was taking care of her she thought I was her mother. She suffered and had a slow death and today I wish I knew how to cope with Alzheimer's better. It could almost have been enjoyable, because I believe people with Alzheimer's disease can be taught again just like a child, if people were only educated about the disease and what changes to expect. One of the things I learned is the part that music, children and pets play in making a person with this disease respond in an enjoyable way. My son who loved his granny so much spent a lot of time playing his guitar and singing to her and she would sing with him — she was happiest at those times.

Because looking after my mother made me aware of the large amount of elderly people and the lack of services, I started a group to meet these needs. We provide day care for the elderly to take care of all their needs and am happy to say on the 30th October 1997 this group said this would not have happened but for my dearest friend, my mum, who I loved and love forever.

We will always remember her as the most gentle, most caring, and loveable mother and grandmother and friend - her name is Chrissie.

Letter to Mama

Dear Mama

Looking back it's hard to figure when it all started, you were such a gentle mother.

I remember you collected loads of unwanted shopping and walked out of the shop without paying. It was lucky I was with you,

you only laughed and said 'you were slowly going around the bend'. I did not think much about it at the time as you just seemed to be a little absent-minded.

There was also lots of other times when things were not right eg. when you went to Mass with your slippers, the time you put the tea in the kettle, burnt the dinner, forgot messages and the time you gave £50 to the coal man and thought it was £20 and the time you put the toilet paper in the fridge and the food in the bathroom.

If I only knew then what I know now. You eventually became very withdrawn so we decided to take you to the doctor. He told us you were suffering from depression, he said 'we should take you on holiday'. We took you on holiday but this confused you more. One day you came to the shopping centre with me and I told you to sit down while I did the shopping. I was only gone for a few minutes and when I came back to ask you something you were gone. I searched the centre and eventually found you with a shop assistant and she was very confused as she couldn't understand what you were saying to her. This really upset you. I scolded you like I would a child. If only I knew at this stage what was wrong!

We took you to another doctor. He asked you to tell him the names of your grandchildren — you gave me a hurt look — then you called out your own children's names. We were told you had Alzheimer's disease, and when we told you, you said in your usual assuring voice, 'Don't take any notice of him'.

The saddest thing is looking at photographs of you at my daughter's wedding. You dressed up in a hat and suit, a lovely looking woman with a vacant look in your eyes, where previously, I would have seen such a proud expression. If I only knew you didn't know what was happening.

What were you thinking Mama? Where was your mind? You seemed to age suddenly in mind and body.

We took you for a brain scan only to be told that all your cells had died off. How confused you were — putting your clothes on over your night-dress, putting both your feet into the one leg of your tights.

If I only knew as much as I do now when you got your stroke, I prayed you would live. I took you home and exercised your arms and legs until you were able to move normally again. Looking back I wish you had died then at least you would have died with dignity and I would be left with little guilt, but because I didn't know about this dreadful disease Alzheimer's, I did a lot of wrong things which to this day I will always feel guilty about. The only thing I feel good about is you were here with me and you were loved so much.

Mama, I miss you so much, but because of you, you being such a caring person and having loved the elderly, I have continued to make some effort to make life easier for the carers and elderly. While you were with me, I started a group and over the years we have worked hard to build a Day Care Centre so that the elderly will be better cared for. In some ways your illness is now helping others. Still I will always regret not knowing enough about this disease Alzheimer's. Educating people will make life better for the sufferers and carers.

Always loved and never forgotten

Your loving daughter Mary

Alzheimer's disease came by stealth: *Jane Webborn*

Mary is a trained nurse and worked in nurse education for many years. Most of her experience is with children's nursing which she enjoys. A year ago Mary left her job, rented out her house, and moved into the loft conversion of her parent's house. Mary had last lived there twenty-eight years ago as a teenager, now she wanted to support her mother in caring for her father. He had first shown signs of dementia seven years previously when he was sixty-four years of age.

Alzheimer's disease came to the family by stealth. John's parents had both died before retirement age with no obvious neurological problems. John had six children with his wife Frances and the family were close and in the phase where grandchildren were growing in numbers. Sharing the joys of young families was a huge pleasure for the proud grandparents. Christmas gatherings were times of happy chaos, and cooking for twenty-two was normal, with everyone lending a hand. It had always been open house with daughters-in-law mucking in. Long walks on wintry beaches were balanced by evenings of telling stories, watching television, or games with the younger ones.

All this began to change in a subtle way and although the adult children were busy getting on with their own lives they began to notice something was wrong with their father. John had been successful as a businessman and at sixty had set up his own consultancy work. He also chaired meetings of various societies within his professional sphere. He attended conferences and kept a high profile with many business colleagues. Slowly he was losing his grip but overcame this in may ways, for example by borrowing notes from colleagues to write up his minutes. A couple of car accidents followed longer journeys and lost wallets were fairly frequent. However, life was very full and concerns did not seem to weigh too heavily, John's nature was happy-go-lucky.

A turning point for the family came when a game of charades went very wrong. It was New Year's Eve and three of the children were working on film and book titles for the game. When it came to John's turn to act out the symbols of the film title there was a long silence. Amongst laughter and encouraging noises John simply said 'I can't do this' and walked out of the room. This was totally out of character and the children and their wives looked around at each other. It seemed to confirm some unspoken fears that all was not well. A curtain seemed to be coming across which had been clear from the look of confusion which covered their father's face. This could be what Is called the invisible side of Alzheimer's, but the incident passed and nothing else abnormal happened.

Sometime later Mary was visiting the family home when John wished to make a phone call. He looked at the push buttons and lifted the handset. After a pause he said 'I can't use this' and left the address book open next to the phone. Mary did not offer to help as he had not asked. The reality of the problem seemed very clear but it was not yet time to take over. The knowledge Mary had as a health care professional made her recognise the fact that the cognitive task of choosing the numbers when displayed on the phone was too much for her father. It caused her some pain and yet she was not able to offer help. Her denial of what was happening, was not in relation to the inability to make a phone call, it was more the denial that the start of a progressively more caring role was needed.

Trips to the general practitioner (GP) and later referral to a centre for a CT scan revealed an overall healthy man except for enlarged ventricles. It was indicative of Alzheimer's at the age of sixty-six.

Frances accepted that the outlook was not good, but at that time the impact was subtle and, there was a drug available which was then on trial. Before embarking on this route, Mary went with her parents on a holiday to Petra in Jordan. The trip was undertaken on the basis that it was worth doing whilst it was possible to do so. Everything went well however, John's fine co-ordination movements were not good enough for him to use a camera. Other than this, he was able to cope with the coach trips, long walks around historic sites and the company of the tour group. His sentences were fairly short and he struggled for some words. The caring role at this time involved packing for him and taking charge of the money, tickets and time schedules.

One incident showed Frances that her husband was coping with the changes he was experiencing in a silent and solitary way. A long morning flight found John looking for a toilet, but on finding one he came out looking worried and said 'I'll just have to bear it'. Despite this stoical approach Frances found that when he had dressed that morning he had put his boxer shorts on the wrong way round. The inability to problem solve was clear but so was his determination to keep up appearances. Mary shared a few glances with her mother and later tears of grief that he was slipping way. In the midst of the beauty of ancient art and culture there was no escape from the reality of the tragedy unfolding before their eyes.

Next came the reading of textbooks on Alzheimer's, trying every sort of remedy and co-operating with medical and mental health staff. Each member of the family had a theory and it seemed helpful to air these between themselves — 'Hadn't Dad been taking lots of aluminium in an anti-acid preparation for reflux?' 'Didn't he spend long hours inhaling glue solvents as he busied himself with his hobbies of making up aeroplane kits?' None of these theories changed anything but there was a strong desire to lay the blame somewhere.

In addition John's son Mark told the others of a dream he had had of the old days. It was then important to hold on to the memories of when John had been the father who had been so full of life. He had a way of making things happen combined with a sense of fun and he encouraged reasonable risk taking. He was the driving instructor to most of his children and gave confidence and encouragement without criticism. He borrowed equipment from a work project and taught his eldest daughter, Morag, to use an aqua lung. His outlook reflected his belief that the world was a good place. In addition to this, he had inherited his mother's spirituality and simple faith, which was at an emotional level more than an intellectual level.

Other family members had dreamt too. Mary had a dream where she was intensely angry at her father, working with a sense of rage. Frances dreamt that John was restored to health as she asked him 'what was it like not being able to communicate?' Even without deep analysis it seems that dreams help bring about a degree of resolution or at least resignation. In Alzheimer's there is so much conflict. The role of carer means that the carer's own needs are not heeded; often by the very person who had done so for many years before. The struggle to keep the cared-for clean, well fed, amused and warm begs the question 'how long for?' It is good to acknowledge that from time to time the carer thinks 'all this tender care will keep him going longer and mean I will have to do this for longer.' 'The release of death could be hoped for, not only because the cared-for would not suffer any more or slip further into a passive, disabled role, but because the carer has had enough. To think this way caused great conflict as the spouse remembers wedding vows, promises to stick together through rain or shine. The loveliness of both partners becomes apparent, each hanging on as best they can.

John had great respect for doctors and submitted to their wisdom. He surprised Mary one day by taking her aside and holding her hand. 'I have Alzheimer's' he said. She hugged him and it was never mentioned again. Mary heard from her brother that he had also been told something we had known for at least a year. He stopped driving at this time.

The forerunner of 'the trial drug' did no good and began to give gastric side effects. There was no wonder drug to help and the disease process had gone too far.

Gradually more and more was added to the list of tasks shifted from John to his wife. The managing of the house and finances, planning the weeks and months to arrange some diversions, and things to look forward to. It seemed as though the world was slowly closing in. Travel abroad seemed too daunting for all concerned but, at the age of sixty-seven, John managed the trip to Jersey with his wife and Mary. By then country walks were daunting, and he would often say, 'how will I get back?'

Mark combined travel to North America with a holiday for John and a convention with his work. They visited Morag, the eldest daughter who had lived abroad for many years. Morag had wanted to get her father over one last time. He had visited before on business and they had shared memories of those trips. To Morag this was a reminder that she had left parents in Britain and time did not stand still and it meant she would now travel back more frequently to follow the grim progress ahead.

Frequently when they met, John's children would wonder 'will I get it too?' Those bouts of forgetfulnesses jump out and wave a flag which says 'Alzheimer's'. The sorrow for John is mixed with the possible, anticipated sorrow for themselves. Mark's wife would joke of her determination to help him make an end if he became too disabled. Black humour also extended to some of John's behaviour. Frances would say she needed to laugh occasionally. It seem healthy because it meant she had not forgotten that there was another normality out there where people were independent and caring was at an emotional level more than at the toilet, fastening a seat belt, organising false teeth in their pot at night.

Family members enter into a more intense dynamic and what was strong before will hold, but any rifts will deepen, under the pressure. John had accepted his disabilities and sometimes even his passive submission to help could be aggravating. The child-like approach made him a bundle of need. When his needs were met he could mix in social company and, at a superficial level, people might hardly notice especially as Frances filled in gaps in conversation. John always recognised people he knew but after the first 'Hello, I'm very well' was at a loss, old friends enjoyed a hug rather than words from 'John'. It seemed things could play on his mind about the past. 'George' he would repeat from time to time days after his old friend had rung to say hello.

As the burden of caring grew heavier other carers were employed in the house. At the first John objected and if this persisted the carer was discontinued. One older woman Peggy was slowly taken to heart though. John enjoyed walks to the park and together they looked at the shrubs and occasionally pinched cuttings. Peggy's blood disorder meant she could not continue and, when she died, John and Frances attended the funeral. Even after two years John would point to shrubs in the park and say 'Peggy' with warmth and sorrow in his voice.

John does not seem typical in his path through Alzheimer's. His strength of emotional connection with people and his faith are very powerful. The net outcome is the same as far as the family are concerned. Here is a man with severe disabilities who needs care input which drains his nearest relatives to unimaginable degrees.

Section under the Mental Health Act — Linda's story: *Elizabeth Robinson*

At the age of 81 years, Mrs Jones was sectioned under the Mental Health Act in February 1997, following domiciliary assessments by a community consultant psychiatrist, two approved social workers, and the general practitioner. The diagnosis which was made for the first time was Alzheimer's disease. Her primary carers for many years were her younger son, Peter and daughter-in-law Linda. Occasional respite breaks were made by her elder son, John in order to allow Peter and Linda to go on holiday. Until then, it had been assumed that Mrs Jones was suffering from senile dementia which had been the general practitioner (GP) diagnosis.

The disease progression followed on from a long-standing history spanning at least 25 years of manic depression (again retrospectively diagnosed) and for which Mrs Jones had on numerous occasions sought, accessed, occasionally accepted and then refused to accept consistent treatment from her GP. She had repeatedly refused psychiatric referral. This pattern of behaviour was translated into the family's 'struggle' to ensure that Mrs Jones received appropriate care. The aim was to provide for her needs within her own home for as long as possible, where she felt most secure and which was close to where Peter and Linda lived. It was anticipated that as her condition deteriorated help would be utilised from a variety of private and social service agencies in order to meet Mrs Jones' needs and lend support to family carers.

Mrs Jones had been a committed mother to her children and in her professional life worked as a schoolteacher. She was very interested in the development of children whom she loved and seemed to have a special understanding. She was also a political activist. Mrs Jones was fiercely independent and stubborn, highly intelligent, talented, creative and caring. Psychologically, her health status was impaired by a recurring pattern of marked mood swings with phases of hypomania, reflected in animated and hyperactive but productive behaviour and awful depressions which made her 'take to her bed'. Her personal appearance and her home were immaculate. The aim of the family was to attempt to maintain integrity in the continuum between who she had been and her changing personality.

The disease progression until the section under the Mental Health Act spanned from 1989 to 1997.

Following the death of Mr Jones in 1988, Mrs Jones' mental health was assaulted by the grieving process, a natural response to loss, but complicated by her pre-existing poor mental health status. A marked deterioration in her mental and subsequently physical health ensued. The family linked this change specifically to a shoplifting incident in the local chemist's which led to her being arrested and cautioned by the police. Although Mrs Jones 'begged' the police that her son not be informed this was quietly done. As far as possible Peter and Linda escorted Mrs Jones on shopping trips to the high street and took her on supermarket shopping trips. Over time, Mrs Jones became canny and adept at 'stealing', even in the presence of relatives. The family responded as far as possible in a low key manner, either by placating shopkeepers or making a decision not to return goods because of the need to protect Mrs Jones from the implications of discovery, thereby minimising any trauma to her from the shame she would feel. Her confidence in shopping never returned, and this coupled with increasing short-term memory loss, resulted in her frequently visiting her local newsagents in the same day for her newspapers, which had been delivered and the post office for her pension, when she had received it. She frequently lost her pension book, along with car and house keys. At times even if 'lost' items had been recovered, she would ring Peter and Linda to say that they had been lost again, sometimes on several occasions on the same day.

The memory loss was always evident when talking to family members and topics were repeated again and again within each hour. Initially, this could be altered by stimulating Mrs Jones to talk about things of interest to her which required long-term memory, for example, her school-teaching career, and items from history or politics. As the illness progressed, stimulation became increasingly problematic and recognition of family members receded.

She was unhappy to engage in any social activity unless it was with family with whom she felt 'safe'. She enjoyed family meals, rides out in the countryside and going to the cinema with Linda. The latter often involved some difficulty whilst Mrs Jones 'settled down' to the film plot. She usually engaged in loud disapproving commentaries in the early stages of a film which could be embarrassing and disruptive. She was particularly disapproving of the language in 'Four Weddings and a Funeral' and at each church service she let the whole cinema know that she thought 'sacrilege' was being committed. Linda weathered these episodes with gentle coaxing which usually worked. At the end of every film outing Mrs Jones always proclaimed loudly how much she had enjoyed the event.

When out in public Mrs Jones greeted strangers as if they were long lost friends and was particularly affectionate and effusive with children and babies. This sometimes provoked confusion in the recipients and alarm from the mothers of children. Peter and Linda always sought to distract Mrs Jones' attention on such occasions by pointing out other things in the environment and gently steering her away from these focal points of her interest.

Additionally, increasing loss of bodily functions, for example, bladder control, occasionally subjected Mrs Jones to the embarrassment of incontinence in public.

Towards 1997, such outings became impossible on a regular basis due to Mrs Jones' deterioration.

Mrs Jones became a hoarder particularly focusing on money, which was found in numerous places, handbags, notepaper, purses and sunglasses. The latter items looked new on discovery and the family could not always be certain how she had come by them. They could only maintain a close watch when she was taken out and distract any unhelpful behaviours but this did not take into account the periods of time when they were not present. She liked to fold up numerous pieces of tissue or roller towel repetitively and put them away in various drawers.

An annual holiday away with John, the eldest son, and family became impossible because Mrs Jones began to pace all night long and create noise and disruption. She was always disorientated if she slept away from home. Additionally, when spending time at Linda and Peter's home, she would after a while become restless and ask to 'go home'. Towards 1997, on each occasion she would make this request very shortly after arrival. She only seemed to feel totally secure in her own home environment.

Self-neglect followed with personal hygiene limited to washing her hands and face and refusing to wash further or be helped to bath even with the gentlest of coaxing. She wore the same clothes daily, refusing to change them or choose immaculate, matching sets as she had always done previously. Clean clothes could become soiled in a short time. Basic household tasks were left, for example, in one day the toilets and kitchen could become quite filthy. Any suggestion or move from family to work 'with' Mrs Jones in carrying out household tasks was met with aggression, anger, or some form of hostility when even the gentlest approach was used. The same response occurred through attempts to ensure nutritional needs were met. Mrs Jones went from preparing simple meals, to eating foods prepared by Linda, to not eating food prepared, to eating pounds of biscuits. She always ate heartily with family but neglected herself once alone even when meals were provided. She refused 'meals on wheels' and these were abandoned.

Similar neglect was mirrored in her treatment of the cat on whom she doted but who she refused to allow out or permit Linda to put a cat-lit tray (attempted on numerous occasions) in the house. Consequently, the cat defecated or passed urine in the house in a specific corner or on a specific chair which was cleared up every day by family members. Sometimes she would wrap up the cat's faeces in tissue paper and throw it out of the bedroom window.

Linda and Peter responded to the difficulty of Mrs Jones' hostility to help by subterfuge. Regularly, Peter would take Mrs Jones out shopping or for a drive whilst Linda blitzed every aspect of the house, clothes and bedding washing. Fresh clean replacements were made and clean day and night clothes put out. New laundry was subtly returned. It was rare for Mrs Jones to comment on changes in the household when she returned. She usually maintained that she had carried out the housework herself but if she had any awareness that Linda or Peter had been involved she would become irrationally angry. Helping was always construed as confrontation.

On the nutritional front, favourite foods were identified and strategically placed in containers in the kitchen and fridge. The main staple diet apart from meals with the family were biscuits, bananas, chicken pieces, tea, milk and fruit juice. Mrs Jones also liked favourite sweets.

The cat became neurotic because of its imposed limitations, in spite of daily feeding by Peter or Linda, who tried to regularise its life but with great difficulty. Latterly, Mrs Jones took to wandering at night-time around the block with the cat on a makeshift lead. At other times she would wander in her night clothes. Neighbours expressed concern and some were quick to criticise not realising the extent of the family input. No one offered to help except Mrs Jones' next-door neighbour who promised to contact the family by phone if she was unduly alarmed. Linda requested help from the GP on several occasions but the response was that there was very little available support on the NHS. She began to lose awareness completely and walk around the garden or inside the house partially clothed and leave the electric hob turned on, on the stove. Even with gentlest of coaxing she would refuse help.

Attempts to introduce nursing support to be alongside Mrs Jones and to maintain the house with the additional support of a cleaner were thwarted. Mrs Jones refused to allow strangers inside the house. Linda and Peter continued to respond to her needs through subterfuge but were becoming worn. Linda had the additional concern that Peter became seriously and chronically ill during 1993–1997 and the situation with Mrs Jones was becoming clearly untenable. Previous attempts to gain medical support had been thwarted by Mrs Jones who had refused admission to the house by the domiciliary consultant psychiatrist and also the GP on more than one occasion.

Following a family discussion with the GP in January 1997, it was decided to refer Mrs Jones for a domiciliary psychiatric visit at which Linda and the elder son John would be present.

The account of the psychiatric assessment and resultant management of Mrs Jones will now be told by Linda herself.

Linda's story

I was at my wit's end and exhausted by the time the consultant came to see Mum. I did not know how I was going to carry on without getting Mum extra help or rather helping her to see that she needed it. I was worried that my health would fail and then there would be nobody to look after anyone. I was dreading the doctor's visit in case mum would not let him in. If she became angry I knew that nothing would be achieved but my brother-in-law wanted to be present and he said he would make sure the doctor got inside the house.

On the day of the visit, Mum wore a jumper, pants and tights and had washed her hands and face and combed her hair. In spite of the absence of her skirt she looked quite presentable. As usual, I tried to get her to put more clothes on but she was adamant that she was fully dressed.

The doctor arrived and the consultation took place with the four of us present in the room, Mum, my bother-in-law, John and myself. I thought this was a break through in a way because she stubbornly refused to allow us usually to be present at any doctor consultations.

I told the doctor mum's history, our original aim in caring for her and all our attempts to meet her needs. I felt such a failure because it didn't sound as if we had done either much to help her and what had been done wasn't good enough because it wasn't helping her condition. I felt guilty during the conversation because it seemed pathetic that two of us between ourselves had put so much in but without much to show for it. The doctor remarked to mum how nice the house was but that I was getting tired. Mum said that she did all the housework and shopping. She showed no awareness of my role and when asked she did not know who I was, although she knew my face nor did she recognise John.

I asked the doctor if there was a possibility of mum ever accepting help from anyone else and he said it was most unusual 'in these cases'. I then asked him what his opinion was on mum's diagnosis. 'Alzheimer's', he replied.

I was shocked and at the same time relieved because although I did not know what this meant it was something concrete. Sometimes I wondered if we were imagining how serious mum's condition appeared to be and especially because we had come to accept her behaviour and it was a kind of 'normal'. I asked the doctor what could be done if mum would not be helped because I was worried about my husband's health and I did not know how long I could go on. He replied so insensitively: 'We can't "section" your mother-in-law just because you're tired.' I was mortified. I burst into tears and left the room. John tried to be supportive of me to the doctor whilst I composed myself. I explained to him that the last thing that we wanted was for mum to be forcefully admitted to hospital, it had never been in our plan of caring for her. We had hoped to achieve everything within the home. The doctor claimed that it was rare to have to section an elderly person in these circumstances. I later found out that this was not true. At the end of the assessment, he informed us that he thought mum was a 'borderline' case and he would invite an approved social worker to come and make an assessment the next day. If she were in agreement he would sign the forms so that mum could be admitted to hospital for assessment and treatment. He explained that a third signature indicating agreement had to be gained from the family GP for the legal process to be completed. I felt devastated that it had come to all this but at the same time I felt insecure because if the other professionals did not think mum was too bad I did not know where else to go for help.

The next day two social workers did an assessment on mum but they did not want us to be present. At about 4pm the same day, I received a phone call from the approved social worker, Christine, to tell me that they had completed the assessment, signed the forms and referred to the GP for her final assessment and signature. She told me that she did not know how we had coped for so long and that even if mum had agreed to accept more care at home social service could not provide the care we had given. I wept with relief and guilt. Relief that at long last someone who could help us believed us and guilt over the type of hospital admission. I must have cried and talked to the social worker for about twenty minutes on the phone.

The GP agreed with the assessment and signed the form. Three signatures were now obtained and mum's hospital admission to the mental health unit would go ahead the following day. The GP rang my husband at 10pm that night as she was having doubts over her decision over the type of admission. I could hear the conversation and I felt dreadfully worried. My husband spent about thirty minutes reassuring the GP that the right decision had been made. I felt confused and doubting which meant I had a sleepless night wondering whether or not the decision would go ahead. However, the approved social worker with a colleague admitted mum for assessment and treatment as planned the following day. This was the first occasion that it had been possible for mum to receive any thorough medical care since her deterioration.

I continued to feel relieved for many months, that other people were now involved in her care and guilty that her life had taken this direction in what seemed like something out of a Dickens novel. But at that time I did not know anything at all about Alzheimer's disease. Visiting her in the mental health unit was so traumatic because we always dreaded leaving her, she wanted to come with us, we didn't know whether or not to just take her and the way she got upset was like a child when it cries, 'don't leave me, Mummy'. The guilt and sadness in these moments was dreadful. It has never really left me, but Peter must feel worse than me, she is his mother.

We have feelings too: *Anonymous*

I never thought of myself as a carer, but have certainly learned to be a more caring person as a result of being faced with the responsibility of looking after an elderly mother who has an increasing need of support. I don't think I used to care a great deal when she first began to be forgetful. All too frequently I would remark, 'you've already said that' when she repeated the same thing for the umpteenth time. I regret my impatience now but didn't realise then that it didn't matter what she said. She just needed a sympathetic, listening ear.

Although her deterioration has been gradual I think that looking back over the whole process there have been a series of stages or steps, when I have realised that since she was not managing to care for herself in some respect, some adjustments needed to be made to the level of support that I was providing. As she has become slowly more dependent on me and I have increased the level of support I have given, we have become closer both literally and metaphorically. Literally in the sense that I have learned to feel more sympathy and love for this person, who has become increasingly dependent on me as if she were my own child, instead of the other way round. (In fact she sometimes even calls me 'Mum'). Metaphorically, in the sense that as she has gradually lost her autonomy, I have learned to interpret her personal needs and feelings when she has been unable to express them herself. As I have tried to understand and meet her needs she has surrendered all responsibility for making decisions about her life to me.

I think I am particularly fortunate, that despite the constant deterioration in her ability to undertake the routine day to day aspects of caring for herself, she still continues to live independently with the assistance of a range of support services for the elderly. Her autonomy has been eroded away to the point where she depends on her instincts and inherent determination for survival, but the habits of a lifetime are so ingrained, that she still seems to be able to manage some of the basic routines that are part of an independent lifestyle.

With my support, and intervention when I believe it to be necessary, a kind of equilibrium has been achieved that could be described as a state of reasonably good health.

Until her early eighties she managed to be quite independent, living on her own, as a widow in a flat close to our house. She liked to observe regular routines, collecting her pension on the same day every week and doing a little shopping daily at the local supermarket. One of the first signs I noticed of her later increasing confusion was her difficulty remembering to collect her pension. Her lifetime habit of paying bills promptly and keeping strict control of financial matters began to waver. I became aware that I needed to check carefully whether she had paid her bills at all or even tried to pay them twice. I realised how vulnerable she was, depending on the honesty of the assistant at the local post office to unravel problems of over- and underpayment of bills. Yet I felt reluctant to take over her financial matters entirely, as I knew that it was important for her pride, to try to retain control over her own affairs. I believed that it was necessary to leave her to make decisions about her own life as far as possible in order to retain her autonomy.

The first substantial change in her life occurred when she fell while walking to the supermarket. My daughter who liked to visit her grandmother regularly, found her sitting dishevelled and distressed one evening at home, although she insisted that she was not hurt. Visiting her the next day I realised that she had injured her arm and needed hospital attention. An x-ray at the local casualty department revealed a fracture which by this time appeared to be causing her a lot of pain. However I don't believe that she would have admitted any physical need for help had I not taken the decision for her.

For the first time I needed to assume complete responsibility for her care as her injury prevented her from managing anything without assistance. As I undressed her that evening I realised that she had not been looking after her own personal care very adequately. Her extremely dirty underwear had not been washed, I suspected, for many weeks. It seems reasonable to assume that the urge to maintain personal hygiene and cleanliness is to a large extent socially constructed.

I believe that the problems my mother was encountering, with her increasing confusion, reinforced her already low sense of self-esteem. Probably the happiest period of my mother's life after she had been widowed was when she took an active part in helping me to look after my children. It was a great help to me when I first returned to work to know that my mother was prepared to collect the children from school and give them their tea. The children themselves benefited from being able to build a very close relationship with their grandmother, and for many years after they ceased to need collecting from school, she would prepare a special tea for them on Sundays with a selection of the things she knew they liked most. What subsequently happened to this long-standing family tradition is a sad reflection of the failing abilities that made it increasingly difficult for her to maintain her perception of being able to perform a useful function in our family life. She continued to bake cakes for the Sunday tea until her late seventies. These were supplemented by home-made sausage rolls and dishes of set custard left over from her Sunday lunch (she was always a good cook). Although the home baking was replaced by shop bought goods by the time she reached her early eighties, she still continued to make small dishes of custard, as these were a particular favourite of my, by then, teenage children.

To help my mother manage the food preparation, that she was finding increasingly difficult, I began to prepare extra amounts of the meals that I cooked for my family to freeze for her use. I also shopped for her and stocked her fridge and freezer at weekends when I was not working. However the logical process that was involved in remembering to defrost portions of food and then reheat them was too much for her to manage. The meals remained in her freezer untouched. Frequent checks of the contents of her fridge revealed out-of-date and unopened packets of food. I began to wonder if she was eating anything in the week apart from biscuits. Any discussion about whether my mother had noticed that a particular food needed eating produced the predictable response: 'I'm saving that for tomorrow'. I finally decided that a change in arrangements was needed when I found portions of the food that I had prepared for her, growing mould in a cupboard where she had placed it, rather than the fridge where it belonged. I felt that it would be so easy for her to contract food poisoning if she subsequently ate any forgotten food that it presented a possible danger to her health.

Her social life had always been centred on her own family. Although she was acquainted with a number of people in the neighbourhood she had no real friends. Once she was confined to her own home no one visited her apart from me and my immediate family. Her natural reluctance to go to any organised clubs or events was compounded by her increasing sense of lack of self-worth. Asked if she would like to go to a particular event, her usual reply was, 'No, I might make a fool of myself.'

Quite a period of time elapsed before my feelings of concern about my mother's needs caused me to discuss her situation again with her GP. She was becoming increasingly insular, often choosing not to attend her luncheon club which remained the only way she was ever able to go out independently. It was often very difficult to obtain any response as a result of ringing her doorbell and I would find her sitting crying on many occasions when I arrived at her flat. Her voice seemed to have lost any expression and her appearance was increasingly uncared for. The only clue as to whether it was her degenerative condition that was causing her deterioration or an emotional reaction to the changes that she was experiencing, was her response when asked what was worrying her: 'I didn't know being old would be as bad as this.'

Her memory of events in her life was so limited at this stage that she lived in the present. There was no possibility of a sense of accomplishment, or satisfaction, by reflecting on the happier moments in her existence because she did not remember anything that she had done in the immediate past.

She was able to dress herself in the morning without any help but seemed to forget to brush her hair which usually looked very dishevelled. When I decided to comb it thoroughly for her one day it was so matted that I realised that she probably hadn't brushed it through for months. Sometimes it was difficult to judge when it was time for me to take a more active role in a particular aspect of her care. It seemed important to preserve her sense of dignity by allowing her to manage as much of her own personal care as possible but there was a risk that my reluctance to assume control of a certain area of her life could cause me to neglect a real need for help.

I think that the quality of the relationship that exists between the carer and person who is being cared for is an important factor when judging the fine balance that exists between infringement of dignity, and neglect of real need. However the existence of a close relationship does not ensure that the choice will always be made correctly. Even though the cognitive functioning of my mother was impaired, and she was not as concerned about the reactions of others as previously, she still had an awareness of her own person-hood and was capable of feeling embarrassment and shame. These feelings arose both from her sense of her own inability to control the rising tide of her confusion and her refusal to acknowledge that she needed any help at all. It was so easy also for me to assume when looking at her blank, increasingly expressionless face, that she did not care about what was happening to her.

I consider that I am fortunate to be able to continue to work to meet the demands of a family and a time consuming job. This causes me some guilt when I reflect on the problem that I don't have enough spare time to provide the constant companionship that would help to meet the mental health needs of my mother. I believe that I am putting my own mental health needs first, asserting my right to lead a rich and fulfilling life (while giving her as much care as I possibly can) until further changes in her condition, which are bound to occur, make it necessary to adjust again the level of support that I provide. It's all a very complicated balancing act.

Appendix
Where to get help

The following information applies to Britain only.

If you are caring for a person with dementia you will eventually need help, however well you are coping at the moment. Services are available from your health authority, your social services department and from some voluntary and private organisations. Your role as a carer is now recognised by law, and you have a right to ask for the service you need. Sharing the care from an early stage will give time for the person with dementia to get used to different arrangements. It is better to be prepared than to leave things until a crisis, when the person may find it hard to adjust.

General practitioner (GP)

If someone appears confused or forgetful or behaves in a way that seems out of character, the first person to contact is the person's GP. It is important to do this quickly as there are a number of treatable conditions and certain prescription drugs which can cause these symptoms. Once these causes have been ruled out, the GP will usually refer the person to a specialist for a diagnosis. You can ask for a referral if the GP does not suggest it. None of the forms of dementia is medically treatable, but continued contact with the GP is essential as he or she will be familiar with the person's medical history, can keep track of their condition and will know about services available in your area.

Specialists

A consultant is a doctor attached to a hospital department or clinic with specialist knowledge in a certain area of medicine. If a person is suspected of having dementia, they may be referred to one of a number of specialist consultants:

- a **neurologist** is a specialist in disorders of the brain and nerve pathways
- a **geriatrician** is a specialist in the illnesses suffered by older people
- a **psychiatrist** is a specialist in mental iness
- a **psychogeriatrician** is a specialist in mental illnesses of older people.

One or more of these doctors may work together in a specialist clinic.

Other medical professionals

As there is no straightforward test for dementia, a number of different medical professionals may help to assess the person's condition. These professionals may also be involved in providing ongoing advice and support. They may be based in a hospital department or clinic, or they may be able to visit the person at home.

- a **clinical psychologist** helps to assess memory and other mental skills and offers appropriate support
- an **occupational therapist** advises on aids and adaptations and on ways of helping the person to retain their living skills
- a **physiotherapist** advises on suitable exercise for people at all stages of dementia, and can also give advice on safe ways of lifting and supporting them
- a **speech and language therapist** helps to assess the person's speech and advises on ways to improve commnication.

Keeping well

It is especially important for a person with dementia to keep in good general health. Problems with eyes, ears or teeth, for example, will only add to their confusion and communication problem. Your GP can refer the person to any or all of the following services:

- an **audiologist** tests hearing and can fit a hearing aid if appropriate (these are provided free on the NHS)
- an **optometrist** carries out eyesight tests and also checks for signs of glaucoma, cataracts, hypertension and diabetes. A person with dementia may be entitled to a free test and help with the cost of glasses (see page on welfare benefits)

- a **chiropodist** looks after a person's feet, which is essential for maintaining mobility.

The person or their carer should also contact their dentist so that any major treatment can be carried out as early as possible. The community dental service can refer you to an NHS dentist who understands dementia and will be willing to make home visits.

Community nursing

A person with dementia may be referred to services which provide nursing support at home (these are often attached to a GP surgery or clinic, or you may be able to contact the community health council direct):

- **community psychiatric nurses** (CPNs) support people with mental health problems, their families and carers. They carry out home assessments and advise on behavioural difficulties and ways of caring. They will not normally carry out practical nursing tasks
- **district** or **community nurses** help with such tasks as dressing, bathing and supervising medication. They can also advise on equipment and aids
- **health visitors** offer advice on benefits, services and voluntary organisations, suggest ways of helping the person with dementia stay healthy, and offer support to both the person and their carer
- most GPs also have **practice nurses** who can carry out nursing tasks at home, advise on aids and equipment, help cope with incontinence and sometimes provide counselling and emotional support.

Social services department

The social services department will be listed in the phone book under the name of the local authority. It is important to contact them as soon as dementia is diagnosed as it can take time for services and support to be organised. A social worker will usually be assigned to assess the person's needs and decide — in consultation with the person him- or herself and their carer — what services are appropriate. Social workers can also advise on benefits and can offer emotional support and counselling if you want to talk things through. You will be given a care plan outlining the help the department agrees to arrange, and this should be reviewed regularly with the carer and the person with dementia. The services may be provided by the local authority or — increasingly — by other voluntary and independent organisations, who have to meet recognised standards of care. The person with dementia will also be assessed for the amount they can contribute towards the cost of their care. If you disagree with any of these assessments, you should seek advice from the Alzheimer's Disease Society or your local Citizens Advice Bureau (see below).

Services available

- A **home help**, sometimes called a **home care** or **community care assistant**, can offer practical assistance with light housework, shopping, cooking, and more personal care such as dressing and supervising meals.
- A **care attendant** offers a similar service in a very flexible way to allow respite to carers. They may sit and chat, take the person out and help with personal care tasks outside normal working hours.
- **Meals on wheels** provide a hot meal daily.
- A **continence adviser** advises on dealing with incontinence and may be able to offer useful aids. There may also be an incontinence laundry service in your area.

Your GP or social worker can advise on any other local services that may be available.

Carers

- The **Carers National Association** is the national voice of carers in the UK. Its work involves raising general awareness of the needs of carers and providing information, advice and support. After campaigning for the Carers' Act which, since 1 April 1996, has given carers legal recognition, it is now monitoring its implementation. The Association also successfully campaigned for the invalid care allowance to be paid, when necessary, to married women (previously it was only available to married men) and has won important council tax concessions for carers.
  The Association is constantly pressing for the level and scope

of financial support for carers to be reviewed, and strongly believes that carers who want to continue in paid work should be encouraged to do so. To this end it works in partnership with several major companies, such as British Gas, offering advice and training on developing care-friendly policies. The Association receives some government funding, but seven per cent of its income is raised from voluntary donations.

The Carers National Association's booklet, *Take Care of Yourself*, is available free as part of a special information pack. Write to:

Carers Information Pack
20–25 Glasshouse Yard
London
EC1A 4JS

You can also get expert advice by ringing the Association's helpline on: 0345 573369 (Monday to Friday, 10am – 12 noon; 2pm – 4pm. Calls are charged at local rates).

- **The Princess Royal Trust for Carers**, telephone: 0171 480 7788, has a network of 65 carers' centres across the UK providing support, information and practical help.
- **Crossroads Caring for Carers**, telephone: 01788 573653, provides respite care.

Independent organisations

Services to people with dementia and their carers are often provided by voluntary groups or private agencies. You may be able to contact these directly through your GP, through your local Alzheimer's Disease Society branch or group or through your local Citizens Advice Bureau. Make sure that any service you use is registered with the social services department, which means that the standard of care has been examined and approved. If you find yourself paying for a service that you need, contact the social services department and ask if they will help with the cost. Often voluntary groups also run day centres, lunch clubs, respite care schemes and support groups. They may offer information, equipment loans and help with transport. A self-help group will give you the advice and back-up that you need, and can tell you about services available through self-help or voluntary organisations in your area.

- **The Alzheimer's Disease Society** offers up-to-date advice on the help that you can expect to receive. You can contact them at:

10 Greencoat Place
London
SW1P 1PH

or by phoning the Alzheimer's Helpline on: 0845 300 0336. Local branches of the Society also run many services including day care and respite care.

- **Age Concern** publishes a list of fact sheets and books on all aspects of caring. For a catalogue, telephone freephone: 0800 009966 (Monday to Sunday, 7am – 7pm), or write to:

Age Concern
Freepost (SWB30375)
Ashburton
Devon
TQ13 7ZZ

Age Concern's experts are also available to give advice and answer questions on a special helpline, telephone freephone: 0800 7314931 (Monday to Friday, 9.30am – 5pm). For people with hearing loss who have access to a textphone, the number is: 0181 679 2832.

Other useful contacts

- **Age Concern England**
268 London Road
London
SW16 4ER

Tel: 0181 679 8000

- **Association of Crossroads Care Attendant Schemes**
10 Regent Place
Rugby
Warwickshire
CV21 2PN

Tel: 01788 573653

- **Citizens Advice Bureau**
Look in the phone book for your local branch.

- **Help the Aged**
  St James's Walk
  London
  EC1R OBE

  Tel: 0171 253 0253
  Free advice line: 0800 289404 (10am – 4pm weekdays)

- **MIND (National Association for Mental Health)**
  Granta House
  15–19 Broadway
  London
  E15 4BQ

  Tel: 0181 519 2122

- **CANDID** (at the National Hospital for Neurology)
  2 Neurosurgery
  Queen Square
  London
  WC1N 3BG

  Tel: 0171 829 8772
  Fax: 0171 209 0182

- For further information about younger people with dementia, the **web address** is: http://dementia.ion.ucl.ac.uk/candid

- **Email**: info@alzheimers.org.uk

This information was prepared by:

> **The Alzheimer's Disease Society**
> Gordon House
> 10 Greencoat Place
> London
> SW1P 1PH
> *Tel:* 0171 306 0606
> *Fax:* 0171 306 0808

How to contact the Alzheimer's Disease Society

Your first call should be to your local branch – look up Alzheimer's Disease Society in the phone book. But if you cannot find one, call the Alzheimer's Helpline, or your regional office:

- **Alzheimer's Helpline**, telephone: 0845 300 0336
- **Email**: info@alzheimers.org.uk

Regional offices

There are over 300 branches and carers' support groups around the country. To get details of what help is available in your area, contact your nearest Alzheimer's Disease Society regional office:

Northern
Yorkshire
Trent
Mersey and North West
Midland
Eastern
London
Southern
South West
Wales
North Wales office
Northern Ireland

Northern

(Cleveland, Cumbria, County Durham, Northumberland, Tyne and Wear)

Alzheimer's Disease Society
The Bungalow
Sheriff Leas
Springfield Road
Newcastle-upon-Tyne
NE5 3DS

Tel: 0191 271 4040
Fax: 0191 271 2233
Email: 101660.2150@compuserve.com

Yorkshire

(Humberside, North Yorkshire, West Yorkshire)

Alzheimer's Disease Society Yorkshire Regional Office
The Retreat
Heslington Road
York
YO1 5BN

Tel: 01904 431265
Fax: 01904 431257
Email: 101660.2153@compuserve.com

Trent

(Derbyshire, Leicestershire, Lincolnshire, Nottinghamshire, South Yorkshire)

Alzheimer's Disease Society
Stonegravels House
Sheffield Road
Chesterfield
S41 7JW

Tel: 01246 557370
Fax: 01246 556421
Email: 101660.2172@compuserve.com

Lincolnshire office
Alzheimer's Disease Society
Wellington Hall
Wellingore
Lincoln
LN5 0HX

Tel/Fax: 01522 811732

Mersey and North West

(Cheshire, Isle of Man, Lancashire, Manchester, Liverpool)

>Alzheimer's Disease Society
>Healey House
>Withington Hospital West
>Didsbury
>Manchester
>M20 2LR
>
>*Tel:* 0161 448 2039
>*Fax:* 0161 448 7457
>*Email:* 101660.2171@compuserve.com

Midlands

(Hereford, Worcester, West Midlands, Shropshire, Staffordshire, Warwickshire)

>Alzheimer's Disease Society
>Drawbridge House
>44A Worcester Road
>Bromsgrove
>Worcestershire
>B61 7AE
>
>*Tel:* 01527 871711
>*Fax:* 01527 870771
>*Email:* 101660.2163@compuserve.com

Eastern

(Cambridgeshire, Essex, Norfolk, Suffolk)

Alzheimer's Disease Society
Abbey House
30 Angel Hill
Bury St Edmonds
IP33 1LS

Tel: 01284 725045
Fax: 01284 725052
Email: 101660.2165@compuserve.com

Central

(Bedfordshire, Berkshire, Buckinghamshire, Hertfordshire,
Northamptonshire, Oxfordshire)

Alzheimer's Disease Society
16 North Bar Street
Banbury
Oxfordshire
OX16 0TF

Tel: 01295 273401
Fax: 01295 275724
Email: 101660.2170@compuserve.com

London

(London, Middlesex)

Alzheimer's Disease Society
45–46 Lower Marsh
London
SE1 7RG

Tel: 0171 620 3020
Fax: 0171 401 7352
Email: 101660.2174@compuserve.com

Southern

(Dorset, Hampshire, Isle of Wight, Kent, Surrey, East Sussex, West Sussex, Wiltshire)

> Alzheimer's Disease Society
> 90B The Street
> Ashstead
> Surrey
> KT21 1AW
>
> *Tel:* 01372 276989
> *Fax:* 01372 274857
> *Email:* 101660.21@compuserve.com

South West

(Bristol, Cornwall, Devon, Gloucestershire, Somerset)

> Alzheimer's Disease Society
> 11–15 Dix's Field
> Exeter
> Devon
> EX1 1QA
>
> *Tel:* 01392 274327
> *Fax:* 01392 274235
> *Email:* adsexeter@compuserve.com

Wales

> Alzheimer's Disease Society
> Tonna Hospital
> Neath
> West Glamorgan
> SA11 3LX
>
> *Tel:* 01639 641938
> *Fax:* 01639 639608
> *Email:* 101660.2157@compuserve.com

North Wales office

Alzheimer's Disease Society
2 Glanrafon
Bangor
Gwynedd
LL57 1LH

Tel: 01248 353608
Fax: 01248 353605

Northern Ireland

Alzheimer's Disease Society
403 Lisburn Road
Belfast
BT9 7EW

Tel: 01232 664100
Fax: 01232 664440
Email: 101660.2161@compuserve.com

Index